MIKAYLA FIT

MikaylaFit Foods

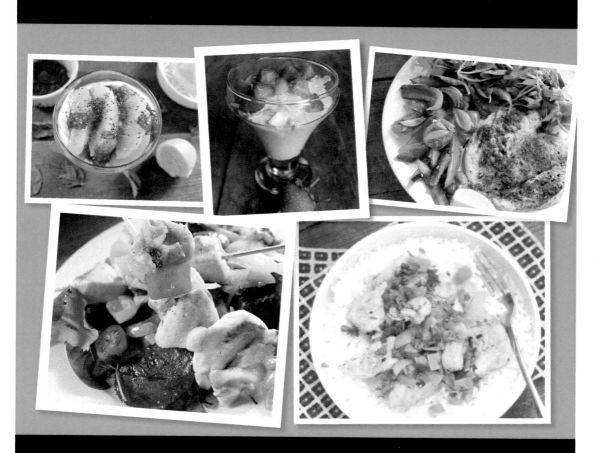

100 Healthy, Easy, Macro Friendly Recipes

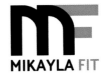

Medical Disclaimer

Always consult your medical practitioner, registered dietician or nutritionist before making any significant changes to your diet – particularly if you are an adolescent, pregnant, breastfeeding or have or develop a medical condition.

Whilst our recipes can help most people lose weight as part of a calorie controlled diet and active lifestyle, they have not been specifically designed for you and individual results will vary.

Where calorie and macronutrient information is provided, it is calculated using common databases. Exact values will vary, however, and so the values will only be approximations for your finished dish.

Image credits (Hormone guide section):

Breakfast cereal: ifong©123RF.com; Snack bar: Baiba Opule©123RF.com; Sandwich: Sara Winter©123RF.com; Cookies: Mariusz Blach©123RF.com; Pasta Bake: Elena Veselova©123RF.com; Refined carbohydrates: akz©123RF.com; Sunshine: Nicola Zalewski©123RF.com; Sleeping Lady: Valeriy Lebedev©123RF.com; Chocolate Dessert: Elena Veselova©123RF.com

Contents

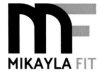

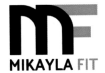

MIKAYLA FIT

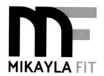

MIKAYLA FIT

Lunch

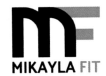

MIKAYLA FIT

Dinner

About me

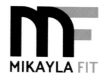

Mikayla Custance is a published fitness model and seasoned figure competitor, gracing the stage in several national and international events annually, a certified fitness nutrition coach, certified physique and figure specialist and personal trainer.

She started out riding horses at just 9 months old in her home town, Gibsons, on the Sunshine Coast. As she got older, her love for equestrian competition ignited the drive to be the best. She competed in 3 day eventing, and as a result, at 16 years old, Mikayla's mom hired a personal trainer to improve her overall strength, conditioning and endurance to ensure a more competitive edge at her events. It was this very training that ignited within her a love and passion for fitness.

At 17 Mikayla stepped on stage for the first time and hasn't looked back! What began as a tool to help her own athletic performance turned into a thriving career as the owner of MikaylaFit to help others improve their health with weight-loss, physical longevity and athletic performance.

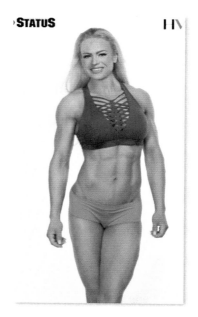

Meet our nutrition team

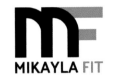

Alan Carson is a contest prep coach and world class physique competitor / bodybuilder. He founded Fitpro Recipes with Naomi in 2012 after realising that nutrition was a common stumbling block for personal training clients. Alan understands the importance of being able to dial in nutrition to get results. He also knows knows that enjoying food and 'not feeling like you are on a diet' is vital to a client's adherence and long term success.

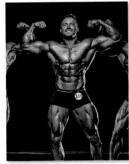

With her experience as a chef, Naomi Carson has been a huge fan of cooking from the moment she was tall enough to reach the kitchen worktop. She knows how to make recipes that taste amazing without taking up all of your time.

Our qualified nutrition consultant Shane Nugent assists with the quality assurance of Fitpro Recipes' products. Shane has helped hundreds of clients and personal trainers achieve their goals through offering world class, science-based nutrition guidance.

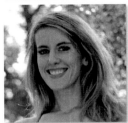

Shane has studied a post-graduate diploma in Sports Nutrition with the International Olympic Committee. He has a masters degree in Applied Sports Science (specialising in Nutrition).

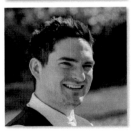

Our passion is food.

We make recipes which are;

- Healthy
- Delicious
- Fat Loss Friendly
- Macro balanced
- Easy and affordable to make

We really hope you will enjoy our recipes as part of your healthy lifestyle and we wish you all the best on the journey that awaits you.

Welcome

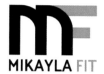

Welcome to MikaylaFit Foods-100 essential healthy recipes! This will be your clean eating bible and go to when you feel stuck on meal ideas!

Nutrition counts for 80% of your fitness results, Which is why I wanted to offer my clients a recipe book full of yummy, easy, clean and healthy recipes. Something more exciting then plain chicken, rice and broccoli!

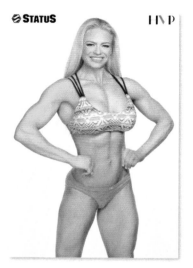

As a certified fitness nutrition coach and competitive figure competitor, I know what to eat and can coach you how to eat, but when it comes to being creative in the kitchen, I'm no expert! So I teamed up with an experienced chef, a fellow competitive bodybuilder and a nutritionist consultant, who has a master's in sports science specializing in nutrition, to bring you 100 clean recipes.

All meals are macro balanced, easy to make, fat loss friendly, healthy and delicious! We hope you enjoy these recipes as part of your healthy lifestyle.

Mikayla Custance

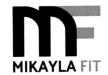

MIKAYLA FIT

Below we have included the key principles that work for nutrition for health and fat loss. If anything you read, see or hear deviates from any of the six principles below, chances are you can dismiss it immediately as a short term fad diet. This is a way of eating that will enable you to achieve both fast and permanent results in a way that is 100% sustainable. You see this change has to be permanent so it has to be both straightforward and above all enjoyable. The good news is that our recipe book will show you how quick, easy and tasty eating this way is.

Follow these principles and you will get results...

1. Eating fewer calories than you burn (calorie deficit)

2. Eat more vegetables and fruits because they are rich in antioxidants and micro-nutrients (vitamins and minerals)

3. Eat plenty of protein for repair and maintenance of lean tissue, and to keep you feeling full (protein satisfies the appetite more than any other macronutrient)

4. Eat enough healthy fats from oily fish, nuts, avocados, coconut and olive oils (healthy fats are an essential part of a balanced diet)

5. Drink plenty of water to naturally detoxify the body, keeping the brain and body hydrated so it can function properly (green and herbal teas count towards this water intake)

6. Limit processed foods and artificial sweeteners and preservatives

Now go and learn, cook, and experience the benefits that our recipes have to offer – enjoy!

Get in touch

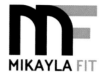

Mikayla Custance

email **mikaylafit01@gmail.com**

f www.facebook.com/mikaylacustancebc

www.instagram.com/mikaylacustance

Let's get started...

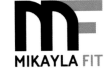

Below are a few hints and tips to help you along the way. I recommend you spare a few minutes to read this before you get cooking.

COOKING WITH FATS AND OILS

Coconut oil, olive oil and ghee are suitable for baking and shallow frying / sautéing. These fats are less likely to oxidise when cooking at medium / high temperatures.

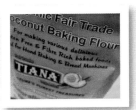

When oils oxidise, they become toxic, which can be damaging to your body.

Coconut oil is high in lauric acid, a fatty acid that is anti-fungal, anti-bacterial and anti-viral.

If you are following a dairy free diet, it is best to cook with coconut oil or olive oil.

When ghee is made, the milk solids are almost completely removed, therefore ghee is often suitable for people who are lactose intolerant.

For salads, use cold pressed extra virgin olive oils, sesame or peanut oils.

COCONUT FLOUR

A gluten free alternative to normal flour. This is a versatile ingredient, which can be used in baking and cooking. Makes great pancakes!

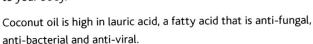

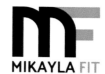

TEA

Green tea has lots of amazing health benefits. It is high in antioxidants and contains about half the amount of caffeine of normal tea. It is widely available in grocery stores, health stores and online.

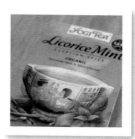

Tulsi Brahmi (caffeine free) is another healthy alternative with healing properties, as well as also being a rich source of antioxidants.

Of all herbal teas, licorice tea is arguably one of the most beneficial yet under-appreciated herbal teas. Licorice tea can help the liver to rid the body of unwanted toxins, can relieve constipation, is used to treat low blood pressure, helps to lower cholesterol and is an anti-allergenic so is helpful for hay fever and conjunctivitis sufferers.

PANTRY ESSENTIALS

There are plenty of simple ways to make your food taste good. Why not keep your pantry stocked up with a handy supply of spices and rubs, which are generally very cheap to buy and a much healthier alternative to the artificial flavorings, additives and sugars found in many of the processed sauces available.

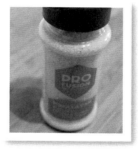

Consider replacing cheap, processed table salt (which is full of chemicals and some even contain sugar!) with a good quality organic sea salt or Himalayan pink salt. This salt contains many beneficial minerals and can help balance electrolytes, eliminate toxins and support nutrient absorption.

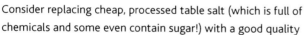

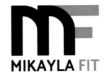

A LITTLE SWEETNESS

Sugar gets a lot of bad press these days due to the negative effects it can have on your health. For example, excessive consumption suppresses the immune system and reduces insulin sensitivity.

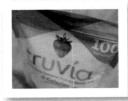

However, we believe it is important to consider the for and against, and not just react to what we see in the news. If you lead a healthy lifestyle, eat a balanced, varied diet, and enjoy moderate regular exercise, then there really shouldn't be cause for panic.

Within the huge category that sugar spans, are a range of good and bad food choices. If, for example, you cut out all fruit for the rest of your life (because fruit contains sugar), you might well miss out on some key nutrients. Plus you may feel deprived.

Our advice to you is that it is your choice if you consume sugar and/or sugar alternatives. But what is probably more important is to consider that worrying about the matter could be equally bad or even worse for your health. Instead, why not try to look at sugar and sugar alternatives as a 'treat' rather than a necessity... something to really savor and enjoy every once in a while (without the guilt!).

In some of our recipes we have used natural sweeteners such as Stevia. Many research studies have been conducted on the safety of these products and while no definite links have been made to any negative health effects, overall the evidence for and against it is still inconclusive. If you'd prefer to swap the sweeteners in my recipes with something else then feel free to do so. Home made apple sauce, raisins and bananas can add enough sweetness to a variety of baking recipes.

Note: There are several forms of Stevia available - a very light powdery texture, and a more granulated/grainy texture. In all of my recipes, we have used the granulated version. We recommend you use the same, so that the ingredient weight is accurate.

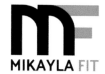

FLAXSEED

Flaxseed is rich in omega-3 fatty acids and fiber. It is a great ingredient to use in cooking and baking, e.g. spelt bread, cakes, pizzas (yes, healthy ones!), mixed in with nut butter or humous dips, added to pancake mixes, sprinkled over cereals or salads or added to smoothies.

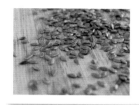

It's best to grind the flaxseed up in a coffee grinder first, as it is not absorbed by the body if left whole. If you mix flaxseed with water and leave to stand for 10 minutes, it develops a sticky coating, which makes it a great egg substitute in baking (as do chia seeds). Always store your flaxseed in the fridge in an airtight container.

WHITE OR WHOLE GRAIN RICE?

Generally speaking, whole grain, unprocessed carbohydrates tend to be better handled than processed carbohydrates such as white rice, pasta, bread and cereals.

Whole grain rice is probably a healthier option than white rice, nevertheless it should still be consumed in moderation, especially if you are trying to lose fat. In most cases, where rice appears in this book, we haven't specified white or whole grain rice. Please decide for yourself which is the best option for you.

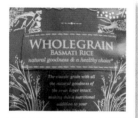

A helping hand...

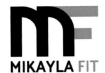

MIKAYLA FIT

Through a combination of good nutrition and exercise, the following recipes will help you achieve optimum fat loss results.

Here are some **low carb recipes**, ideal for a **non training day**:

Breakfast
- Meat & nuts
- Bacon & egg frittata
- Poached salmon protein brunch

Lunch & Dinner
- Turkey coconut burgers
- Low carb quiche
- Crunchy mackerel salad
- Low carb chilli cheese burgers
- Quick fish stew

Snacks & Treats
- Protein-rich Scotch eggs
- Pistachio & goji bark

Smoothies
- Supreme green smoothie
- Pina colada

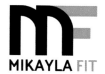
MIKAYLA FIT

Research has shown that the body can tolerate carbohydrate better after exercise. If you are going to consume carbs, you should aim to do this within 2 hours of exercise.

Here are some recipes which are ideal post-workout. These are also medium / high protein to aid muscle repair.

Breakfast
- Fruit & nut porridge
- Breakfast burrito
- Summer fruit pancakes

Lunch & Dinner
- Lentil pepper soup
- Authentic curry
- Chilli con cauli
- Fragrant fish soup
- Warming stew

Snacks & Treats
- Flaxseed spelt bread
- Carrot & ginger loaf
- Indulgent cookie cakes
- Banana yogurt

Smoothies
- Beetroot, orange & carrot cooler
- Oaty berry smoothie

Your guide
to Hormones

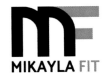

Understanding how hormones work and how our lifestyle choices affect our hormone levels, is vital if we want to get the best results possible. In fact we'd go as far to say that if our hormones are not regulated properly, it can massively sabotage our results and lead to poor health.

Obesity, diabetes and depression are just a few of the diseases that hormonal imbalances contribute towards. Whilst the diagnosis and treatment of hormonal imbalances should be left to medical experts, we can have a positive impact on our hormones by leading a healthy lifestyle.

A basic understanding of the key hormones that regulate metabolism, hunger, body fat, and energy levels is useful for understanding how different lifestyle choices affect your body.

Every time we eat, exercise, sleep, get stressed or meditate; hormones are released.

We want to make sure that our lifestyle choices help us to optimize the way our hormones are working.

What are hormones?

Hormones are chemical messengers that communicate information throughout the body.

You could think of hormones as radio signals that tell different cells in the body to do different things.

Depending on our lifestyle choices, the hormones released will dictate whether we burn or store body fat, feel hungry or satisfied, build muscle or not, feel relaxed or stressed, and whether we are able to sleep well or have restless nights.

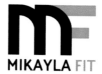

Can you see why this is so important to your health and the results you want to achieve? On the next few pages, we are going to look at a variety of different hormones that influence our health and our body composition. Let's get started...

Insulin

Insulin is released from the pancreas in response to raised blood glucose and increased energy intake. Skimmed milk is more insulinemic than white bread, so insulin is not just a blood glucose hormone. When our blood sugars increase, insulin is released and it's job is to tell the body to store the sugar in our muscles and liver. Insulin transiently inhibits the release of lipids from fat tissue, but even with multiple insulin spikes, energy balance is the sole dictator of fat loss.

To slow the rate in which food leaves the stomach, the majority of our carbohydrate sources should be coming from fiber-rich whole grains. Added sugars offer no nutritional benefits, and so should be minimized but not demonized, as this can lead to poor relationships around food. Insulin's role is to prevent glucose remaining in the blood, as this is toxic. Its role is to move the glucose away from the blood.

The "blood sugar rollercoaster" and the often talked about "crash" is known as *reactive hypoglycemia* and is very rare in non-diabetics. Insulin is actually an anorexogenic hormone, which means it fills you up. Higher insulin releases after meals are associated with increased satiety. This "crash" is often due to postprandial somnolence, which is simply the digestive energy requirement of digesting a large meal. The craving for more sugary food is most likely not due to the drop in blood sugar, but the body craving more easily obtained energy in the form of sugar.

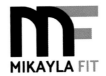

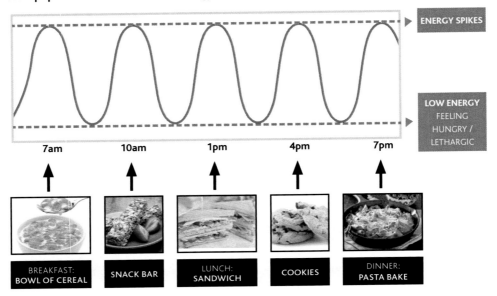

How popular food choices affect energy levels and hunger:

ENERGY SPIKES

LOW ENERGY
FEELING
HUNGRY /
LETHARGIC

7am   10am   1pm   4pm   7pm

BREAKFAST: BOWL OF CEREAL   SNACK BAR   LUNCH: SANDWICH   COOKIES   DINNER: PASTA BAKE

From a fat loss perspective, energy balance should be the key focus. However maintaining good blood glucose control can reduce our risk of metabolic syndrome and diabetes. How well we regulate blood glucose is due to carbohydrate type, fitness level, muscle mass and genetics.

Protein can actually have a higher insulin response than white bread. Both whey protein and skimmed milk stimulate larger releases of insulin. Fiber will slow the rate of gastric emptying and reduce the glycemic load of a meal, while fats on their own, do not raise blood glucose. A combination of carbohydrate and fat will slow down gastric emptying.

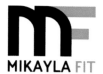

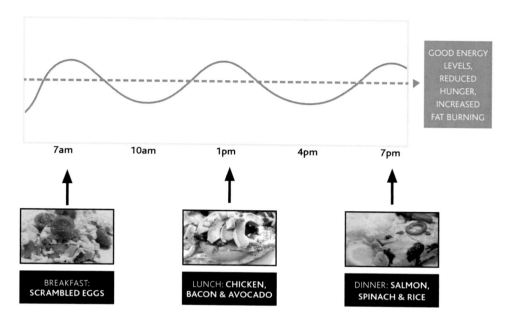

7am	10am	1pm	4pm	7pm

GOOD ENERGY LEVELS, REDUCED HUNGER, INCREASED FAT BURNING

BREAKFAST: SCRAMBLED EGGS

LUNCH: CHICKEN, BACON & AVOCADO

DINNER: SALMON, SPINACH & RICE

Insulin resistance is characterized by either the pancreas secreting too much insulin, or skeletal muscle failing to respond the the effects of insulin. It is a myth that eating too much sugar causes insulin resistance. A cell becoming resistant to insulin is multifaceted and the main culprit is prolonged energy excess in combination with inactivity.

An inactive muscle is less sensitive to the effects of insulin. This can lead to increased likelihood of a build up of serum blood glucose, as the muscle cannot properly utilize the glucose. We then need our pancreas to produce more insulin to shift the same amount of sugar out of the blood and into storage. This can be the beginning of metabolic syndrome and Type 2 diabetes.

The two main culprits behind insulin resistance are a lack of exercise and a hyper-caloric diet high in refined carbohydrates. The good news is that insulin sensitivity can be regained with the right combination of diet and exercise.

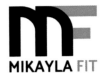
Glucagon

If we think of insulin as a **"storage hormone,"** then we can think of glucagon as a **"mobilisation hormone."**

Glucagon tells our muscle and fat cells to release energy for us to use to fuel our daily activities. If we consume a surplus of Calories and lots of sugary carbohydrates, glucagon doesn't need to do its job, because there's already too much energy available. Insulin and glucagon are both released from the pancreas and work with each other to regulate our blood sugars and energy levels. If our insulin levels are chronically high, this could increase our risk of Type 2 diabetes and metabolic syndrome. When our insulin levels are low, this signals to the body that energy availability is low. If we have poor blood glucose control, this may lead to increased appetite and a sudden urge to eat, which is the reactive hypoglycemia mentioned earlier.

In a nutshell, by eating the right foods to prevent insulin spikes, glucagon can do what we want it to do; help us to use our fat stores for energy.

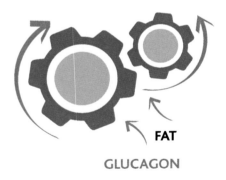

FAT

GLUCAGON

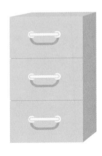

INSULIN

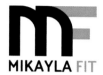

Cortisol

Cortisol is a hormone that is released from the adrenal glands (along with adrenaline). Although cortisol gets a bad wrap, it's actually very necessary for us to have cortisol, just not chronically elevated levels or unhealthy cortisol rhythms.

It's usually described as a stress hormone because we release cortisol (and adrenaline) in stressful situations. If we didn't release cortisol in the morning, then we would struggle to wake up.

Adrenaline tends to be an instant reaction, whereas cortisol works more slowly. Cortisol is a glucocorticoid hormone, so its job is to increase blood glucose to ensure we have an available supply during periods of stress.

Cortisol levels should rise in the mornings so that we feel energetic in the daytime, and gradually lower throughout the day, enabling us to feel relaxed and naturally tired in the evenings.

Modern life can be stressful and if, for example, we are stressing out over a work situation at night, then our cortisol levels can become elevated at a time when they should be low. Overtraining can also cause our cortisol levels to become chronically elevated so it's important that our training programs are assessed regularly.

How healthy cortisol levels look:

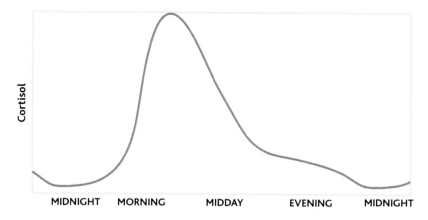

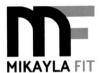

Some of the reasons that our cortisol levels become imbalanced:

- Poor sleeping habits
- Inability to handle or manage stress
- Overconsumption of stimulants; caffeine for example
- Overtraining; training too long / frequently at high intensity

When cortisol gets out of control, we can experience suppressed immune system function, elevated blood sugars, faster ageing and poor insulin sensitivity. This is the perfect recipe for getting sick, overweight and wrinkly. Times of stress often see us reaching for convenient sugary foods that taste good. Stress can often lead to comfort eating, but everyone deals with stress in different ways, so cortisol does not directly cause weight gain, but behaviors associated with stress could.

Things that can help to restore healthy cortisol levels:

- Getting 6-9 hours of good quality sleep every night
- Learning a cognitive strategy such as CBT to learn how to cope better with stress
- Taking time to meditate / relax / chill out more often
- Reducing caffeine intake, especially in the afternoons
- Ensuring your training regimen is assessed regularly

Growth hormone

Human growth hormone has been described as **"the fountain of youth"** and not surprisingly growth hormone supplementation is now big business, especially in the USA. **Good growth hormone levels help to keep us lean, healthy and strong.** As we age, our levels of growth hormone decline. For example, a 60 year old may only produce 25% of the growth hormone of a 20 year old. In that sense, there's not a lot we can do, because we're all getting older. What we can do, however, is to look at ways to help our bodies produce growth hormone normally and naturally.

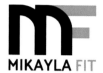

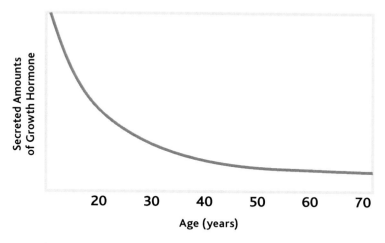

Growth hormone is mainly released / elevated when we are:

- Sleeping
- Exercising
- Fasting

If we are not sleeping properly, not only is our cortisol rhythm disturbed, we also miss out on our natural growth hormone release during sleep. This is another great reason to get to bed early and to watch our caffeine intake.

Exercise causes the release of growth hormones, so if we are exercising regularly then our bodies will be producing growth hormones naturally. Fasting also increases growth hormone levels, which is one of the reasons intermittent fasting has become popular. Whether or not you should fast is an individual decision and it's important to note that although it can increase growth hormone, it can also increase cortisol levels, so if you're already stressed, then fasting might not be the best option.

In terms of muscle gain, fasting is not an anabolic process. Fasting will initiate certain processes in the body like AMPK and autophagy, which are both catabolic clearance of damaged cells and mitochondria. Eating too many sugary carbohydrates can also lower growth hormone, yet another reason to ditch the junk foods.

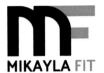

Testosterone

Although testosterone is the dominant male sex hormone, it is produced by both men and women. **Healthy testosterone levels are associated with drive, motivation and virility.** As we age, testosterone production declines and this contributes to the loss of muscle mass that people experience as they age. Low testosterone levels are associated with increased risk of cardiovascular diseases, depression, lethargy and lack of motivation.

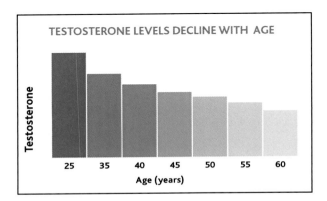

It is to be expected that certain hormones decline with age, in fact it's completely normal and natural, but what is a concern is the generational decline in testosterone levels in males. Our grandfathers, on average would have had much higher testosterone levels throughout their lives.

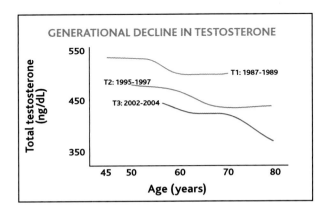

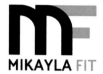

One of the reasons for this is that modern life can be a lot more stressful. So it's not that surprising when we see studies showing that cortisol blocks the effects of testosterone.

What can we do?

Luckily there are things we can do to maintain healthy testosterone levels:

- Get to bed early
- Learn stress management techniques
- Train with heavy weights
- Eat enough fat (our bodies make testosterone from cholesterol)

Training with heavy weights will not cause women to look big and bulky because females have a very small amount of testosterone compared to males, as the table below shows.

TOTAL TESTOSTERONE LEVELS		
SEX	ng/dl	ng/ml
Females	6-86	0.1-1.2
Males	270-1100	1.4-12

This explains the difference in ability between men and women to build muscle mass. It also explains why some men find it easier than other men to build muscle. The normal range has a huge variance, so a man sitting naturally at 1000+ will find it easier to build muscle than a man with low 200s.

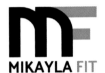

Estrogen

It's often thought that information about estrogen is only relevant to females. Estrogen however, is an important topic for any man experiencing the dreaded "man boobs" or "moobs". **Men need a normal, healthy level of estrogen just as women need a normal healthy level of testosterone.** The problem arises when estrogen becomes out of balance with testosterone. This is when men can literally start growing what look like breasts. Obesity, as well as exposure to environmental estrogens such as plastics, are thought to contribute towards the disruption of healthy sex hormone levels in males.

For women, healthy estrogen levels are essential for heart and bone health, as well as many other functions in the body.

Estradiol is the primary estrogen that a woman relies upon during her younger years to keep her healthy and lean. Estradiol also helps to regulate appetite, mood and energy levels. As a woman goes through the menopause, production of estradiol decreases and this leaves another form of estrogen, estrone, as the main estrogen. Estrone is linked with increased abdominal fat storage and unfortunately, the more fat that is gained, the more estrone is produced. This can make losing body fat much more difficult, and extra attention must be placed upon diet and exercise during and after the menopause. Estrone can also contribute to insulin resistance, another good reason to avoid bingeing on sugary carbohydrates and opt instead for proteins, fats, vegetables and complex carbohydrates.

Estradiol is also vital for calcium synthesis, and this is why women who have been through the menopause will require more calcium.

Another hormone that drops at the menopause is **progesterone**. Because progesterone is a precursor for testosterone and estradiol, this now means that there is less testosterone and estradiol available to have a positive effect on body composition, mood and appetite regulation. This is why it's so important to do everything within our control to promote healthy body composition, mood and appetite regulation. We can do this by paying attention to diet, exercise and stress levels.

email **mikaylafit01@gmail.com** f **mikaylacustancebc** INTRODUCTION 22

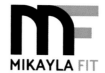

Chronically elevated cortisol levels around the time of the menopause need to be avoided, because cortisol and progesterone may compete for the same receptors. This means that cortisol can exhibit a blocking affect on progesterone. This is definitely not good if we consider progesterone levels are already dramatically lowered after the menopause. **The key message is to learn how to manage stress and make the right lifestyle choices.**

Thyroid

Thyroid hormone is often referred to as "the master hormone" and with good reason. Thyroid hormones have a huge impact on metabolic rate. If you or anyone you know has suffered with under-active thyroid, then you know all about the weight gain and lethargy that can be experienced when the thyroid isn't functioning optimally. On the contrary, when the thyroid is over-active, people lose weight rapidly and can become anxious. **Important nutrients for thyroid health include; iodine, selenium, vitamin D3 and vitamin B12.**

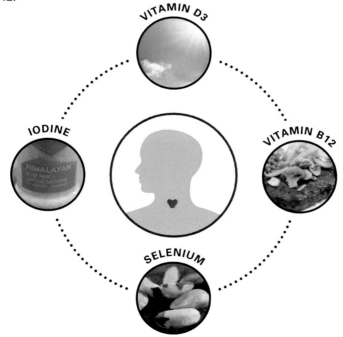

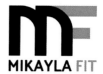

Cruciferous vegetables such as broccoli contain substances called goitrogens that inhibit the thyroid gland. Most of these substances are destroyed by cooking, so it's important to cook your cruciferous vegetables.

Leptin

Leptin is a hormone that decreases hunger by signalling to the brain that we have enough energy (fat) stores in our body. The problem is that, as in the case with insulin resistance, we can become resistant to leptin. The leaner someone is, the more sensitive to leptin they are, so a small amount of leptin does the job of telling us we're not hungry. This makes sense when we consider that leaner people actually have less leptin, even though they have less energy (fat) stored in their bodies.

When someone is leptin resistant, although they may have more leptin, the message doesn't get through and the result is feeling hungry. Not sleeping properly can also decrease leptin levels.

What can we do?

- Take Omega 3 fish oil – Omega 3 fats are associated with decreased hunger
- Go to bed early
- Reduce stress
- Reduce caffeine

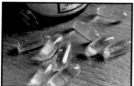 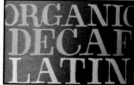 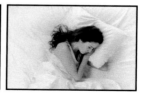

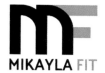

Ghrelin

Ghrelin is the hormone that tells us we are hungry. When it's coming up to meal time, we will naturally feel hungry, because ghrelin is being released. There's not a whole lot we can do to directly influence ghrelin, apart from, you guessed it, sleep well! Studies show that just 2 hours less sleep can increase ghrelin by 27%.

It's not only leptin and ghrelin that regulate our appetite, so we still can put practices into place to help us get our appetite under control.

There are other ways to help:

- Consume fiber-rich foods to help keep us feeling full
- Consume enough protein and fat because these two nutrients help to satiate us more than carbohydrates
- Drink enough water – sometimes when we think we are hungry, we're really just thirsty
- Free sugar containing foods are often not as satiating, so it is likely beneficial to mimimize consumption.

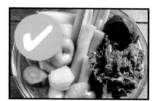
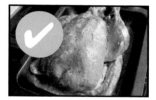
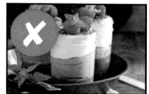

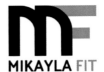

MIKAYLA FIT

Conclusion

There are many hormones in the body, all having unique actions in maintaining sound health. The interplay between all the different hormones is complex, and while we don't need to understand everything about hormones, we can conclude that **the right lifestyle choices play a huge role in balancing our hormones.**

To help balance all of our hormones naturally we need to:

- Ensure that we are getting adequate amounts of good quality sleep
- Learn strategies to cope better with stress
- Taking time to meditate / relax / chill out
- Ensure we are not constantly overtraining
- Perform resistance training
- Reduce caffeine intake

Please be aware that this information does not constitute medical advice. If you are concerned about your hormonal health, please see a qualified medical professional.

Mango, mint & cucumber smoothie

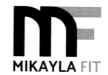

MIKAYLA FIT

1 cup fresh mango, roughly chopped

⅔ cup cucumber

2 cups fresh spinach

1 Tbsp. coconut milk

5 ice cubes

3½ fl oz. cold fresh water

1 sprig fresh mint

READY IN **5** MINUTES

SERVES 2

Put all of the ingredients into a blender and blend until smooth. Add more water if necessary to achieve the desired consistency.

PER SERVING:
81 Calories
16g Carbs
2g Protein
1g Fat

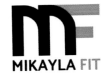

Alkalizing tonic

handful fresh spinach
1 kiwi, halved
2 Tbsps. wheatgrass powder
juice of half a lemon
8-10 fl oz. cold water (depending
on desired consistency)

READY IN 5 MINUTES

Put all of the ingredients into
a blender and blend until
smooth.

SERVES 1

PER SERVING:
121 Calories
20g Carbs
8g Protein
1g Fat

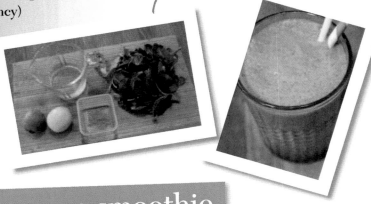

Supreme green smoothie

1 cup spinach leaves
1 Tbsp. fresh ginger,
peeled and chopped
1 tsp. wheatgrass powder
½ cup blueberries
7 fl oz. cold water (add more if
required to reach desired consistency)

READY IN 5 MINUTES

Put all of the ingredients into
a blender and blend until
smooth.

SERVES 1

PER SERVING:
64 Calories
11g Carbs
5g Protein
0g Fat

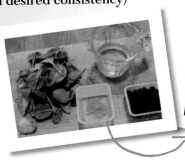

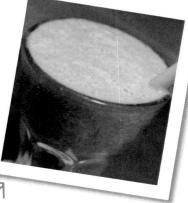

Refresher cooler

4 slices fresh mango
handful fresh spinach
1 Tbsp. wheatgrass powder
handful cucumber, roughly diced
1 kiwi, peeled and diced
2 ice cubes

READY IN 5 MINUTES

Put all of the ingredients into a blender and blend until smooth. Add more water if required to achieve the desired consistency.

SERVES 1

PER SERVING:
109 Calories
21g Carbs
4g Protein
1g Fat

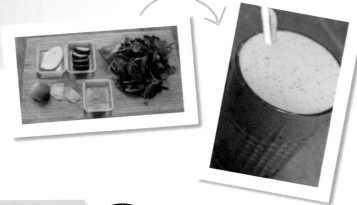

Pina colada

READY IN 5 MINUTES

1 medium sized slice fresh
pineapple, chopped
1 Tbsp. coconut milk
2 ice cubes
3 Tbsps. vanilla flavor whey or rice
protein powder (optional)

SERVES 2

PER SERVING:
145 Calories
7g Carbs
15g Protein
6g Fat

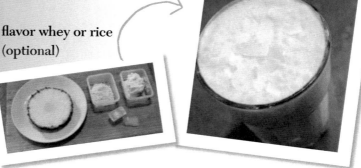

Put all of the ingredients into a blender and blend until smooth.

Beetroot, orange & carrot cooler

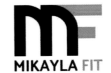

MIKAYLA FIT

2 cooked beetroots
juice of one large orange
3 medium sized carrots,
peeled and cut into chunks
1 tsp. chia seeds (optional)
handful ice cubes
5 fl oz. cold fresh water

READY IN
5
MINUTES

SERVES 2

Put all of the ingredients into a blender
and blend until smooth. Add more water
if necessary to achieve the desired
consistency.

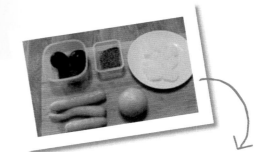

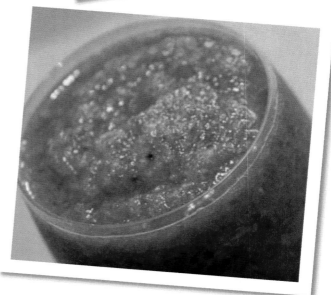

PER SERVING:
97 Calories
19g Carbs
3g Protein
1g Fat

Oaty berry smoothie

MIKAYLA FIT

2 Tbsps. vanilla or strawberry flavor whey or rice protein powder
¾ cup frozen mixed berries
1 Tbsp. porridge oats (use gluten free oats if preferred)
7 fl oz. cold fresh water

READY IN **5** MINUTES

SERVES 1

Put the protein powder, berries and oats into a blender and add half of the water.

Blend together, adding more water until you have the desired consistency.

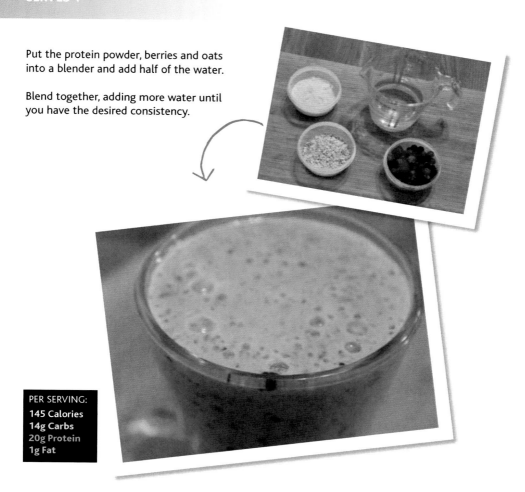

PER SERVING:
145 Calories
14g Carbs
20g Protein
1g Fat

Milk kefir

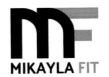

2 Tbsps. Kefir milk grains (available on Ebay or Amazon)
1 x 34 fl oz. glass jar with lid, sterilized
1 x 34 fl oz. full cream milk
plastic sieve
plastic or wooden spoon
glass bottle, sterilised

MAKES 10 x 3.5 FL OZ. SERVINGS

Place the kefir grains in the glass jar. Add the milk and close lid gently (do not close too tightly).

Place jar in room temperature and away from direct sunlight. This is found to be the best environment for kefir fermentation.

Leave for between 12 hours to 2 days. After 12 hours, you will have a mild tasting milk kefir. After 24 hours, it will be more tart. After 48 hours, it will have a more zesty taste.

Use the sieve and spoon to separate the milk from the grains. Pour the kefir milk into a sterile glass bottle and refrigerate.

You can either allow the grains to rest for a few days, covered in a little cold water or milk and placed in the fridge, or start another batch again. Rest the grains every few weeks to get the best from them.

Your grains will last a lifetime, if you look after them!

Note:
Do not allow the grains to come into contact with metal as it will damage them. One shot of kefir milk per day will have a significant impact on your digestive health.

Blend the kefir milk with a handful of frozen berries and a scoop of chocolate flavor protein powder to create a delicious post workout smoothie.

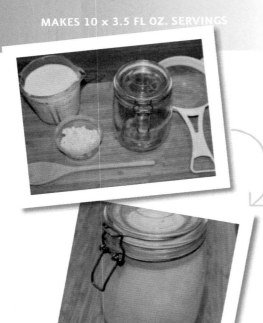

PER SERVING:
81 Calories
5g Carbs
4g Protein
5g Fat

Iced latte protein smoothie

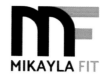

MIKAYLA FIT

READY IN 5 MINUTES

1 small banana
7-10 coffee ice cubes (made with strong caffeinated or decaffeinated coffee)
2 Tbsps. vanilla flavor whey or rice protein powder
5 fl oz. cold fresh water

SERVES 1

Place all of the ingredients in a blender and blend until smooth.

Add a little more water if required, to achieve the desired consistency.

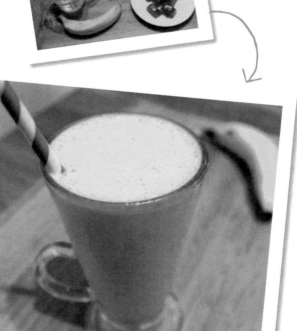

PER SERVING:
218 Calories
25g Carbs
25g Protein
2g Fat

Kale, mint & matcha smoothie

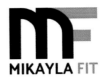

MIKAYLA FIT

6 matcha ice cubes
(see method on right)
1 handful kale
½ cup cucumber, sliced
10 mint leaves
juice of 1 lemon
5¼ fl oz. cold water
1 tsp. honey (optional)

READY IN 5 MINUTES

SERVES 1

How to make matcha ice cubes:

Dissolve 3 tsps. matcha powder in 4.5 fl oz. hot water. Leave to cool then pour into an ice cube tray and freeze

Place all of the ingredients in a blender and blend until smooth.

Add a little more water if required, to achieve the desired consistency.

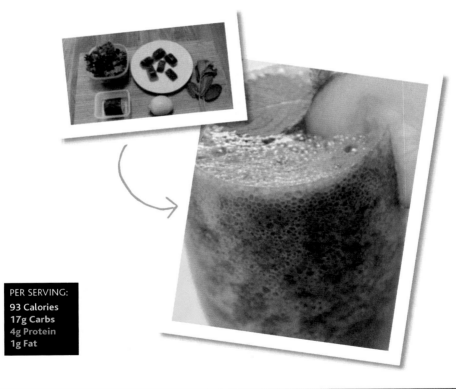

PER SERVING:
93 Calories
17g Carbs
4g Protein
1g Fat

Tiramisu smoothie

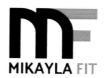

MIKAYLA FIT

1.5 fl oz. strong coffee (use decaffeinated if preferred)
1½ heaping Tbsps. Greek yogurt (use dairy free if preferred)
1 tsp. almond extract
5 fl oz. unsweetened almond milk
½ a small frozen banana
¼ cup vanilla flavor whey or rice protein powder (optional)
1 tsp. cocoa powder
1 Tbsp. cream cheese - optional (use dairy free if preferred)
3 ice cubes

SERVES 1

Place all of the ingredients in a blender and blend until creamy. Serve.

Consume immediately.

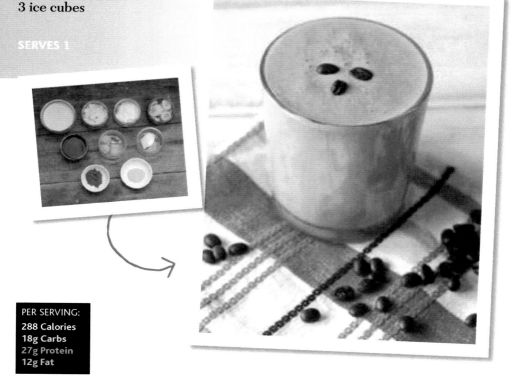

PER SERVING:
288 Calories
18g Carbs
27g Protein
12g Fat

Chocolate figgy bars

¼ cup dark chocolate chips
(minimum 70% cocoa)
1 tsp. coconut oil
⅔ cup dried figs, chopped finely
⅓ cup almond or cashew butter
2 Tbsps. coconut flakes or desiccated coconut
½ tsp. ground ginger
1 Tbsp. coconut oil
2 tsps. chia seeds

MAKES 6 BARS

Line the base of a 6x6 inch tin with baking paper.

Place the chocolate and 1 tsp coconut oil in a saucepan. Bring a shallow basin of water to the boil over a medium / low heat source and carefully place the saucepan in the basin. Stir until melted. Remove from heat and allow to cool for 5-10 minutes.

Mix all of the remaining ingredients in a large bowl until thoroughly combined. Transfer mixture to the tin and spread out evenly. If the mixture doesn't cover the base of the tin, use a spatula to neaten the edges of the mixture.

Pour the chocolate over the mixture and refrigerate until set.

Cut into 6 bars.

Store any leftovers in an airtight container and refrigerate for up to 4 days.

PER BAR:
226 Calories
11g Carbs
5g Protein
18g Fat

Banana yogurt

½ cup plain or Greek yogurt (use dairy free yogurt if preferred)
1 small banana, sliced
1 level tsp. sunflower seeds
1 level tsp. flaked almonds
1 tsp. acacia honey (optional)

SERVES 1

READY IN
5
MINUTES

Spoon the yogurt into a bowl.
Top with the banana, seeds, almonds and honey.

Store in an airtight container and refrigerate for up to 2 days.

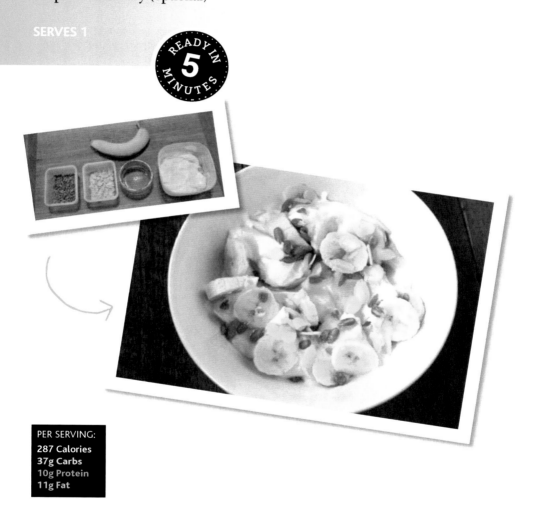

PER SERVING:
287 Calories
37g Carbs
10g Protein
11g Fat

Protein-rich Scotch eggs

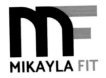

7 medium sized eggs
1lb 5 oz. lean ground pork/
vegetarian alternative*
4 slices lean unsmoked bacon slices,
fat removed, cut into small pieces
(use vegetarian bacon if preferred*)
½ tsp. Himalayan pink salt
pinch of black pepper
1 tsp. dried oregano
4 Tbsps. ground almonds

MAKES 6 SERVINGS

__Note:__ Some meat free alternatives contain gluten and/or MSG. Please check the label before you buy!

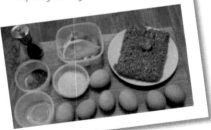

Preheat oven to 150°C/300°F.

Place six of the eggs in a saucepan and cover with water. Bring to the boil, then simmer for 5 minutes. Remove from heat and replace the hot water in the pan with cold water. Set aside.

In a large bowl use your hands to combine the pork, bacon, salt, pepper and oregano.

Break the remaining egg into a separate bowl and whisk lightly. Add a small amount to the pork mixture and mix together.

Cover the surface of a large plate with the ground almonds. When the boiled eggs are cool, peel carefully. Take some of the pork mixture and use your hands to shape it around the egg. Add a coating of the whisked egg to the Scotch egg, smoothing it to help keep the pork mixture in place.

Gently roll the Scotch egg in the ground almonds, until it has an even coating. Place the scotch egg on a baking tray. Repeat the process with the remaining boiled eggs. Bake for 30 minutes.

Store in an airtight container and refrigerate for up to 3 days.

PER SERVING:
267 Calories
1g Carbs
32g Protein
15g Fat

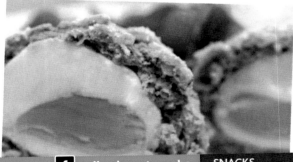

Tri-color energy balls

⅔ cup almonds
½ cup cashews
½ cup pitted Medjool dates
⅓ cup vanilla flavor whey or rice protein powder
2 Tbsps. coconut oil, melted
½ tsp. ground cinnamon
¼ tsp. sea salt
½ tsp. almond or vanilla extract

for the coating:
a sprinkle of unsweetened coconut flakes
2 tsps. ground shelled pistachios
2 tsps. cocoa powder

MAKES 10 BALLS

Place the almonds and cashews in a food processor and process until coarsely ground.

Add the pitted dates. Process again until the dates are finely chopped.

Add the protein powder, coconut oil, cinnamon, salt, almond extract and 1 Tbsp. cold water. Process until the mixture forms a dough. Add more water, 1 tsp. at a time, if the mixture is too dry.

Roll the mixture into 10 balls. Roll each ball in any of the 3 coatings.

Freeze for one hour.

Store any leftovers in an airtight container and refrigerate for up to 7 days or freeze on same day.

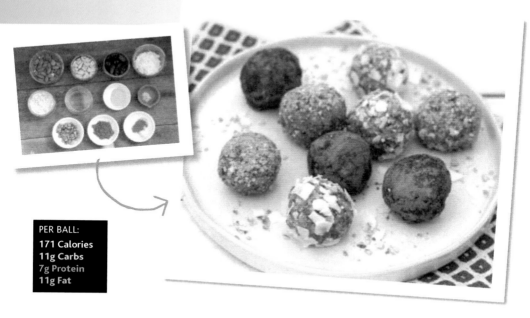

PER BALL:
171 Calories
11g Carbs
7g Protein
11g Fat

Baked onion bhajis

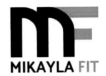

1 cup wheat free gram flour
1 tsp. sea salt flakes
1 tsp. chili powder
1 tsp. cilantro powder
1 tsp. cumin
1 tsp. turmeric
1 tsp. garam masala
3 medium sized white onions, finely sliced
1 medium sized egg
cold water
2 Tbsps. coconut oil to grease tin

for the yogurt mint dip:
1 cup plain yogurt (use dairy free yogurt if preferred)
2 tsps. mint sauce
½ tsp. turmeric
1 tsp. lemon juice
1 tsp. stevia (or natural sweetener of your choice)
small handful fresh cilantro, chopped

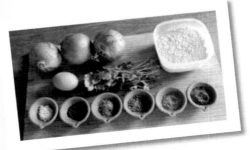

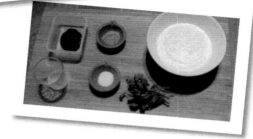

**MAKES 16 BHAJIS &
4 SERVINGS DIP**

PER BHAJI:	PER SERVING DIP:
79 Calories	41 Calories
9g Carbs	5g Carbs
3g Protein	3g Protein
4g Fat	1g Fat

In a bowl, mix the flour with the spices.

Add the flour mixture to the onions and mix well with your hands, squashing the onions as you go, to get the flavor into the onions.

Crack the egg over the onions and mix well for 1-2 minutes, using your hands.

Add a small amount of water and mix well. You'll need a thick consistency and slightly wet but not runny. Add sufficient water to achieve this consistency. Cover and refrigerate for 3 hours or overnight.

Preheat oven to 180°C/350°F.

RECIPE CONTINUED ON NEXT PAGE >>

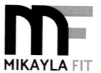
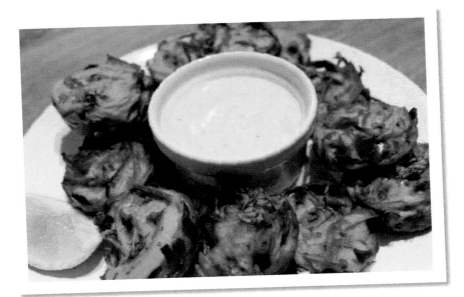

Grease 16 muffin tray compartments with the coconut oil.

Place in the oven until the butter or oil has melted.

Remove from oven, and spoon the bhaji mixture into the compartments.

Bake for around 20-25 minutes, until the bhajis are a golden color and cooked through.

To make the dip: Mix all of the ingredients together. Taste test the dip, adding more lemon or more mint if necessary, according to taste.

Store in an airtight container and refrigerate for up to 2 days.

Fiery fries

2 cups all rounder potatoes
peeled and cut into chips
1½ Tbsps. organic butter or
coconut oil, melted
2 tsps. paprika
good pinch of sea salt flakes
2 tsps. chili flakes

SERVES 2

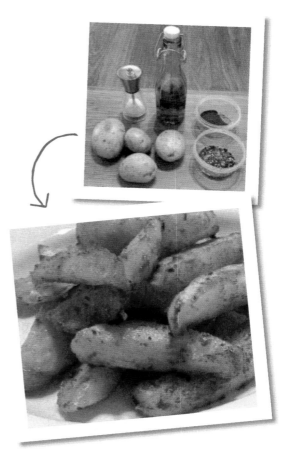

Preheat oven to 170°C/350°F.

Bring a large pan of lightly salted water to the boil. Add the potatoes and cook for around 8 minutes, so that they are still quite firm. Remove pan from heat and drain carefully.

Place a sheet of foil on a baking tray. Drizzle with half of the oil or butter and sprinkle with the paprika, salt and chili flakes.

Add the potatoes and turn over so they get a coating of spices and oil. Drizzle over the remaining butter.

Cook for 20 minutes then turn the chips over. Cook for a further 20-25 minutes until golden and crispy.

Consume immediately.

PER SERVING:
222 Calories
29g Carbs
4g Protein
10g Fat

Creamy banana split

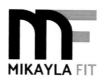

MIKAYLA FIT

½ cup Greek yogurt (use dairy free if preferred)
⅓ cup vanilla flavor whey or rice protein powder
1 small banana, cut lengthwise
½ cup blueberries
4 medium-sized strawberries
½ tsp. flaked almonds
1 square dark chocolate (minimum 70% cocoa), cut into small chunks

SERVES 2

Spoon the yogurt and protein powder into a bowl. Stir well until thoroughly combined. Transfer onto the center of a serving plate.

Place each banana half on either side of the yogurt.

Scatter the berries over the yogurt.

Top with the flaked almonds and dark chocolate. Serve with two spoons!

Refrigerate for up to 3 hours.

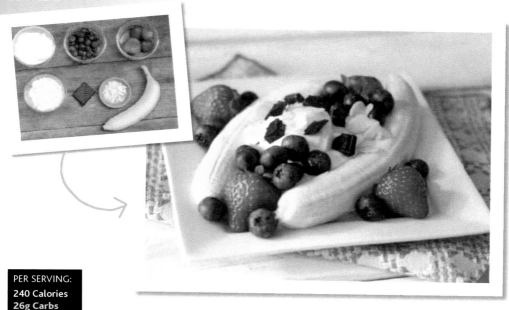

PER SERVING:
240 Calories
26g Carbs
16g Protein
8g Fat

Flaxseed spelt bread

3½ cups whole grain spelt flour
(use gluten free flour if preferred)
½ tsp. sea salt flakes
1 tsp. quick yeast
3 Tbsps. flaxseed
13½ fl oz. warm water
1 Tbsp. olive oil

SERVES 6

Recommended:

Flaxseed is a great antioxidant, rich in
Omega 3 essential fatty acids and fiber

Preheat oven to 200°C/400°F. Line the
base of two medium sized bread tins with
baking paper.

In a large bowl, mix together the flour, salt,
flaxseed and yeast.

Roughly mix the water into the flour.
While the dough is still craggy, add the
olive oil and give it a good mix.

Knead the dough for several minutes, using
a little extra flour to stop it sticking to
your hands.

Divide the mixture into the two bread tins.
Cover with a clean tea towel, and leave
somewhere warm for 25 minutes e.g. next
to a radiator.

Bake for 40-45 minutes. Turn out the
loaves onto a wire rack and allow to cool
for at least 5 minutes before serving.

*Store in an airtight container at room
temperature for up to 3 days.*

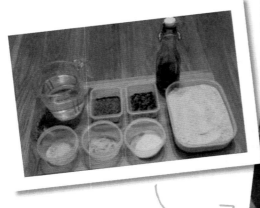

PER SERVING:
331 Calories
54g Carbs
13g Protein
7g Fat

Banana-berry freeze

MIKAYLA FIT

1 banana
3.4 fl oz. cold water or unsweetened almond milk
1⅔ cup frozen raspberries
⅖ cup Greek yogurt (use dairy free yogurt if preferred)
1 Tbsp. acacia honey
few drops of peppermint or chocolate extract (optional)

SERVES 4

Cut the banana into thin slices, and place on a lined tray. Freeze for one hour.

Remove banana from the freezer. Pour the cold water or unsweetened almond milk into a blender and add the banana.

Using a wooden spoon, break up the frozen raspberries into small pieces then add to the blender. Blend on high setting for 3-4 minutes. Add more liquid if the blades jam or leave for 5 minutes for the mixture to soften up, then continue to blend until smooth.

Add honey, yogurt and peppermint extract (if using) and pulse until creamy.

Serve immediately or freeze for a later date. Remove from the freezer 15 minutes before serving.

Refer to your freezer manual for maximum storage times.

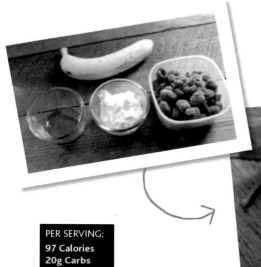

PER SERVING:
97 Calories
20g Carbs
2g Protein
1g Fat

Raspberry protein pudding

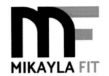

MIKAYLA FIT

⅓ cup oats (use gluten free if preferred)

3 fl oz. unsweetened almond milk (or use milk of your choice)

⅓ cup vanilla or raspberry flavor whey or rice protein powder (optional)

15 fresh raspberries

1 tsp. vanilla extract

a small amount of stevia to taste (only required if not using protein powder. Use an alternative natural sweetener if preferred)

for topping;

5 fresh raspberries

2 tsps. macadamia nuts, chopped

SERVES 1

Mix all of the ingredients in a bowl until thoroughly combined. Refrigerate for one hour or more.

Transfer the mixture to a serving bowl. Top with the macadamia nuts and fresh raspberries.

Serve.

Refrigerate any leftovers for up to 2 days.

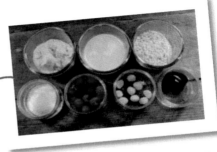

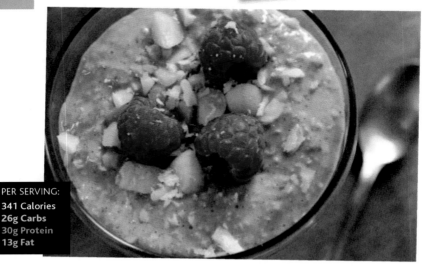

PER SERVING:
341 Calories
26g Carbs
30g Protein
13g Fat

Berry sandwich bars

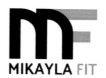

MIKAYLA FIT

¾ cup coconut flour

⅗ cup vanilla flavor whey or rice protein powder (optional)

1 Tbsp. ground flaxseed

½ tsp. baking soda

1½ tsps. cinnamon

½ tsp. sea salt flakes

3 Tbsps. coconut oil, melted

2½ Tbsps unsweetened coconut milk

4 medium sized eggs

2 tsps. vanilla extract

5 pitted dates, finely chopped

2 cups mixed berries

2 tsps. unsweetened coconut flakes

MAKES 8 SQUARES

Preheat the oven to 175°C/350°F. Line a 9x9 inch baking tray with baking paper.

Sieve the flour into a bowl and add the protein powder (if using), flaxseed, baking soda, cinnamon, and salt. Set aside.

In a separate bowl whisk together the coconut oil, coconut milk, eggs, and vanilla until creamy. Add the dates then slowly stir in the flour mixture until well combined and a firm dough forms.

PER SQUARE:
204 Calories
12g Carbs
12g Protein
12g Fat

Divide the dough in half and press half evenly into the bottom of the baking paper lined pan. Spread the berries evenly over top of the dough.

On a separate sheet of baking paper, gently shape the remaining dough into a similar size and shape as before. Lift the dough onto the paper and transfer over the berries like a lid, removing the paper as you go. If it breaks apart, that's fine, just cover the berries as much as possible. Sprinkle the dough lid with coconut flakes, and press lightly to hold them in place.

Bake for 20 minutes, until the coconut is golden and they spring back to the touch. Allow to cool in the pan completely before cutting into squares.

Store in an airtight container and refrigerate for up to 4 days.

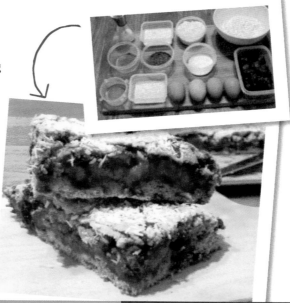

Chocolate & coconut bark

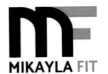
MIKAYLA FIT

⅓ cup coconut oil
3 Tbsps. organic cocoa powder
1 tsp. stevia (or natural sweetener
of your choice)
½ cup chopped nuts
½ cup chocolate flavor whey
or rice protein powder (optional)

SERVES 6

A low carb treat that tastes truly indulgent and will satisfy any sweet tooth.

You can use any type of nuts. Hazelnuts, brazils, macadamias or pistachios work very well. Chop them roughly to add extra texture.

Line a baking tray with baking paper and put in the freezer.

Melt the coconut oil gently in a pan over a medium/low heat. Add the cocoa powder and stevia. Stir well to combine. Remove from heat.

Stir the nuts and protein powder into the mixture. Add a little cold water so that the consistency is thick but pourable.

Remove baking tray from freezer and pour the mixture onto the baking paper, spreading evenly to desired thickness.

Place in freezer on a level shelf and leave for 20 minutes.

Freeze for up to 2 weeks.

PER SERVING:
222 Calories
3g Carbs
9g Protein
22g Fat

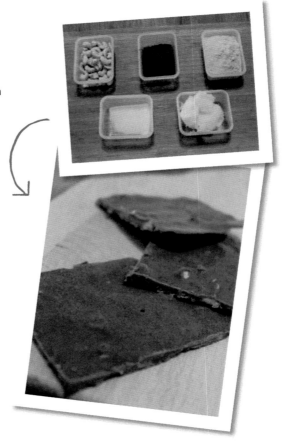

Carrot & ginger loaf

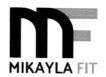

MIKAYLA FIT

2 Tbsps. flaxseed, ground
1 large apple, peeled,
cored and sliced
1¼ cups coconut flour
½ tsp. xanthan gum
2 tsps. baking powder
½ cup chocolate flavor whey
or rice protein powder
pinch of sea salt
2 tsps. ground cinnamon
1 tsp. ground ginger
8 cloves, ground
3 tsps. stevia (or natural
sweetener of your choice)
3 Tbsps. pure maple syrup
3½ fl oz. coconut milk
3½ fl oz. extra virgin olive oil
1 egg
1 egg white
1¼ cups carrots, peeled and grated
½ cup organic raisins
4 tsps. nuts, chopped (any kind)

MAKES 14 SERVINGS

Preheat oven to 180°C/350°F. Line the base of two medium sized loaf tins with baking paper.

Mix the flaxseed with a little water until the consistency thickens. Leave to stand.

Bring a small saucepan of water to the boil. Add the apple and simmer gently for around 4 minutes, until soft. Remove from heat and drain through a fine sieve. Stir gently to remove excess water. Transfer apple to a bowl and leave to cool.

In a large bowl, mix the flour, xanthan gum, baking powder, protein powder, salt, cinnamon, ginger, cloves, stevia and maple syrup.

In a separate bowl, mix the coconut milk, olive oil, egg, egg white, apple sauce until smooth. Gently stir in the carrots and raisins and mix.

Divide the mixture between the two loaf tins and sprinkle the nuts over the top. Bake for 30 minutes. Remove from oven and leave to cool for 5 minutes on a wire rack. Remove from tins and allow to cool.

Store in an airtight container at room temperature for up to 3 days.

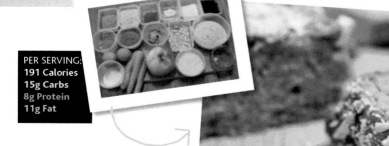

PER SERVING:
191 Calories
15g Carbs
8g Protein
11g Fat

Chocolate nut pancakes

3 heaping tsps. coconut flour

¼ cup chocolate flavor whey or rice protein powder

⅓ cup whole porridge oats (use gluten free oats if preferred)

2 medium sized eggs

1 egg white

1 tsp. cocoa powder

1 tsp. stevia (or natural sweetener of your choice)

4 tsps grated dark chocolate (minimum 70% cocoa)

3 tsps. crunchy peanut butter (no added sugar)

2 tsps. coconut oil

MAKES 5 PANCAKES

Serving suggestion:

Serve with a dollop of Greek yogurt, black cherries (fresh or frozen) and some grated dark chocolate.

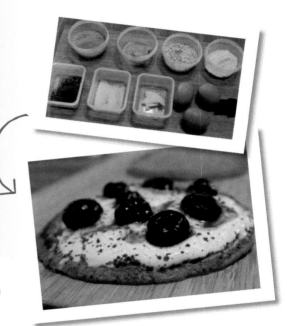

Put all of the ingredients except for the oil into a blender and mix together. Add a dash of water if necessary to achieve the right consistency. The mixture should be quite thick yet runny enough to pour.

Heat some of the coconut oil in a large non-stick pan over a medium/high heat. Pour one quarter of the mixture into the center of the pan.

PER PANCAKE:
148 Calories
9g Carbs
10g Protein
8g Fat

Move the pan around gently to even out the mixture into a circular shape. When small holes appear in the pancake (around 1-2 minutes), turn or flip it over and cook on the other side for 1-2 minutes.

Transfer pancake to a plate. Add more oil to the pan and repeat the process four times with the remaining batter.

Store in an airtight container and refrigerate for up to 2 days.

Cherry almond muffin loaf

MIKAYLA FIT

⅓ cup apple, cored, peeled and sliced
5 medium sized eggs
1 egg white
2 Tbsps. pitted dark cherries, halved
½ cup coconut flour
4 Tbsps. pure maple syrup
1½ tsps. stevia (or natural sweetener of your choice)
½ cup ground almonds
1 tsp. of vanilla extract
½ tsp. baking soda

MAKES 10 SLICES

Preheat oven to 180°C/350°F.

Line the base of a medium sized loaf tin with baking paper.

Bring a small saucepan of water to the boil. Add the apple and simmer gently for around 4 minutes, until soft. Remove from heat and drain through a fine sieve. Stir gently to remove excess water. Transfer apple to a bowl and leave to cool.

Beat the eggs and egg whites with a whisk for 30 seconds.

Add all of the remaining ingredients and mix well. Pour the mixture into the loaf tin and bake for 40-50 minutes, until golden brown.

Leave to cool for 5 minutes, then remove from the tin and transfer to a wire rack to cool.

Once cooled, store in an airtight container at room temperature for up to 3 days.

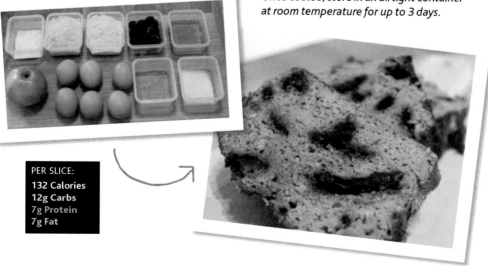

PER SLICE:
132 Calories
12g Carbs
7g Protein
7g Fat

Creamy coconut & strawberry dessert

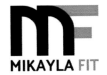

MIKAYLA FIT

⅔ cup Greek yogurt (use dairy free yogurt if preferred)

2 Tbsps. coconut cream (use the fat part from a tin of coconut milk)

¼ cup vanilla or strawberry flavored whey or rice protein powder (optional)

½ cup fresh strawberries, hulled and chopped (reserve a few for topping)

1 tsp. unsweetened coconut flakes

SERVES 1

Place the yogurt, coconut cream and protein powder (if using) in a bowl and mix until thoroughly combined. Stir in the strawberries.

Transfer the mixture to a serving bowl and top with the coconut flakes and remaining strawberries.

Serve.

Refrigerate any leftovers for up to 2 days.

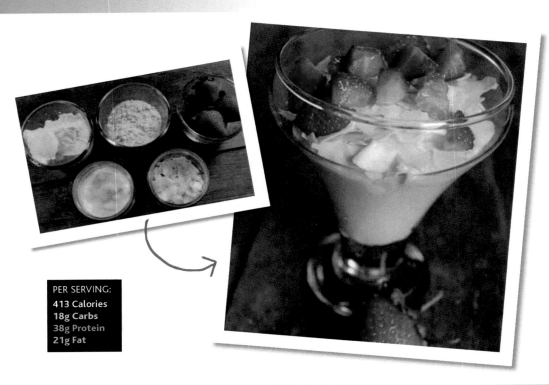

PER SERVING:
413 Calories
18g Carbs
38g Protein
21g Fat

Blueberry bombs

MIKAYLA FIT

2 Tbsps. dark chocolate
(minimum 70% cocoa)
1 tsp. vanilla extract
3 Tbsps. acacia honey
4 Tbsps. crunchy peanut butter
(no added sugar)
1 cup porridge oats (use
gluten free oats if preferred)
2 fl oz. unsweetened
coconut milk
3 Tbsps. mixed seeds (e.g. flaxseed,
sesame seeds, sunflower seeds)
⅔ cup pitted prunes
2 Tbsps. organic desiccated coconut
¾ cup blueberries

MAKES 15 SERVINGS

Put the chocolate in a heatproof bowl.
Pour several inches of boiling water into
a shallow wide based dish. Place over a
gentle heat and allow the water to simmer
gently.

Carefully sit the heatproof bowl in the
shallow dish of water. Melt the chocolate
slowly, stirring regularly. Remove from
heat.

Add the remaining ingredients and mix
well. Refrigerate for several hours.

Roll into 15 balls. Refrigerate until ready
to serve.

*Store in an airtight container and refrigerate
for up to 4 days.*

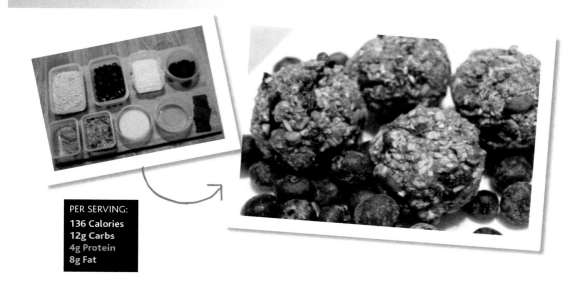

PER SERVING:
136 Calories
12g Carbs
4g Protein
8g Fat

Quick & easy popcorn

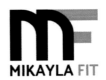

MIKAYLA FIT

½ cup popping corn
3 tsps. coconut oil
sprinkle of stevia to sweeten
(or natural sweetener of
your choice)

SERVES 4

Melt the oil over a medium/high heat in a large saucepan.

Add the popping corn and cover.

When the corn starts to pop, shake the pan gently from time to time over the heat, to prevent burning.

When most of the corn has popped remove saucepan from heat. You will probably find there are a few that remain unpopped. Transfer to a large serving bowl.

Sprinkle on the stevia and mix well.

Consume immediately.

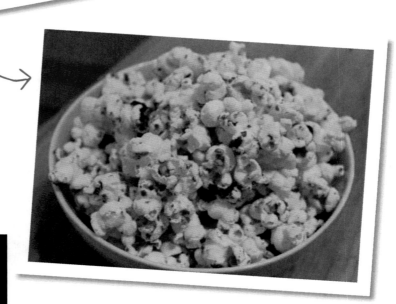

PER SERVING
120 Calories
19g Carbs
2g Protein
4g Fat

Chocolate nut icecream

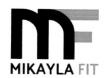

MIKAYLA FIT

⅔ cup 0% fat Greek yogurt (use dairy free yogurt if preferred)
2 medium sized ripe bananas, sliced
½ cup chocolate flavor whey or rice protein powder
1 tsp. vanilla extract
2 tsps. dark chocolate (minimum 70% cocoa), finely chopped
4 tsps. chopped hazelnuts

SERVES 6

Put the yogurt, banana, protein powder and vanilla extract in a blender. Pulse until creamy.

Stir in the dark chocolate and nuts.

Divide into 6 small freezer proof pots.

Freeze for at least 2 hours. Remove from freezer 15 minutes before serving.

Refer to your freezer manual for maximum storage times.

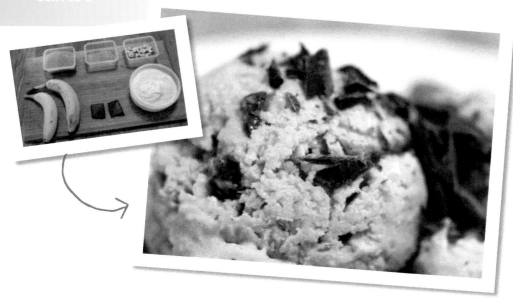

PER SERVING:
156 Calories
14g Carbs
16g Protein
4g Fat

Raspberry & vanilla energy balls

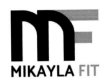
MIKAYLA FIT

⅘ cup raspberries
1 tsp. pure maple syrup (or natural sweetener of your choice)
¼ tsp. ground cinnamon
pinch of nutmeg
1 cup porridge oats (use gluten free oats if preferred)
1 tsp. vanilla extract
⅓ cup pitted dates, chopped finely
¼ cup ground almonds
⅖ cup chocolate or vanilla flavor whey or rice protein powder
8 brazil nuts, finely chopped
2¼ fl oz. unsweetened coconut milk
⅘ cup shredded coconut

MAKES 9 ENERGY BALLS

Pour the raspberries into a fine sieve and position over a large bowl.

Using the back of a wooden spoon, press the raspberries gently, extracting the raspberry juices into the bowl.

Discard the raspberry seeds.

Add all of the other ingredients to the large bowl, except the desiccated coconut. Mix thoroughly and refrigerate for at least an hour until the mixture firms up.

Divide the mixture into 9 portions and roll into balls using your hands. Pour the shredded coconut onto a plate and roll each ball in the coconut, to give them an even coating.

Store in an airtight container and refrigerate for up to 3 days.

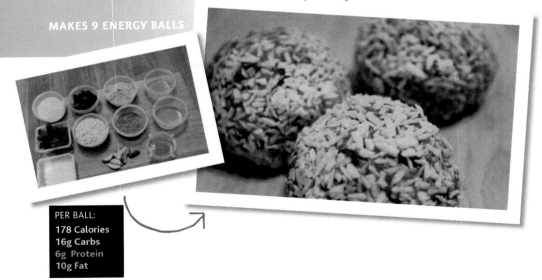

PER BALL:
178 Calories
16g Carbs
6g Protein
10g Fat

Pistachio & goji bark

3 Tbsps. dried goji berries
5 Tbsps. coconut oil
3 Tbsps. organic cocoa powder
1 tsp. pure maple syrup
⅕ cup pistachios, chopped roughly
2 Tbsps. mixed seeds (e.g.flaxseed, sesame seeds, sunflower seeds)
4 tsps. dark chocolate (minimum 70% cocoa), melted

MAKES 12 SERVINGS

Presoak the goji berries in water for 1 hour, then drain. Gently press to remove excess water and chop roughly.

Line a baking tray with baking paper and place in the freezer.

MIKAYLA FIT

Melt the coconut oil gently in a pan over a medium/low heat. Add the cocoa powder and maple syrup. Stir well to combine. Remove from heat. Add a little cold water so that the consistency is thick but pourable.

Remove baking tray from freezer and pour the mixture onto the baking paper, spreading evenly to desired thickness. Sprinkle the pistachios, omega sprinkle and goji berries over the chocolate.

Put the chocolate in a heatproof bowl. Pour several inches of boiling water into a shallow wide based dish. Place over a gentle heat and allow the water to simmer gently. Carefully sit the heatproof bowl in the shallow dish of water. Melt the chocolate slowly, stirring regularly. Remove from heat.

Place in freezer on a level shelf and leave for at least 20 minutes. Remove from freezer 5 minutes before serving.

Store in an airtight container and freeze for up to 2 weeks.

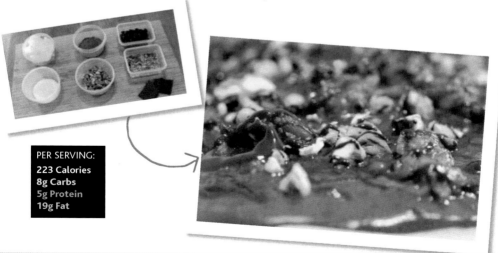

PER SERVING:
223 Calories
8g Carbs
5g Protein
19g Fat

Chickpea cookies

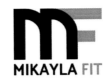

MIKAYLA FIT

¼ cup ground almonds

3 Tbsps. peanut / hazelnut / cashew butter (no added sugar)

3 Tbsps. acacia honey

2 tsps. vanilla extract

½ tsp sea salt flakes

1 tsp. baking soda

1 x 400g can chickpeas, drained

2 tsps. organic cocoa powder

2 Tbsps. dark chocolate (minimum 70% cocoa), finely chopped

MAKES 9 COOKIES

Preheat oven to 170°C/350°F.

Line a baking tray with baking paper.

Mash or blend all of the ingredients (except for the dark chocolate) until fairly smooth.

Spread the mixture onto the baking tray. Sprinkle the dark chocolate over the top and lightly press into the mixture.

Bake for 15 minutes or until a golden brown.

Allow to cool on a wire rack, then cut into 9 squares.

Store in an airtight container at room temperature for up to 4 days.

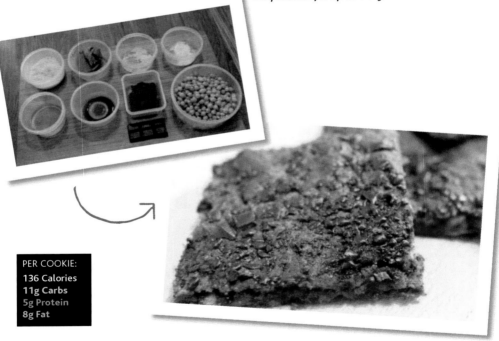

PER COOKIE:
136 Calories
11g Carbs
5g Protein
8g Fat

Berry icecream

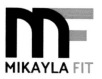

1 cup plain or Greek yogurt (use dairy free yogurt if preferred)
½ cup banana or vanilla whey or rice protein powder
2 cups berries of your choice
¾ tsp. vanilla extract

SERVES 3

Place all of the ingredients in a large bowl and whisk for several minutes until thoroughly combined. It doesn't matter if some of the berries are left whole.

Transfer the mixture to a freezer proof container and freeze for 30 minutes. Remove from freezer and mix thoroughly with a fork. Return to freezer.

Repeat process every 30 minutes a further 2 or 3 times – until the mixture is creamy and resembles icecream.

Remove from freezer 10 minutes before ready to serve.

Refer to your freezer manual for maximum storage times.

PER SERVING:
149 Calories
10g Carbs
25g Protein
1g Fat

Berry protein whip

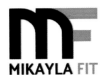

MIKAYLA FIT

½ cup blackberries
½ cup raspberries
⅓ cup fromage frais (use dairy free fromage frais if preferred)
⅓ cup plain yogurt (use dairy free yogurt if preferred)
1 heaping Tbsp. banana or vanilla flavor whey or rice protein powder
½ tsp. xanthan gum (optional)
½ tsp. vanilla extract

SERVES 1

Put all of the ingredients in a large bowl. Using an electric hand mixer, blend the ingredients together for 2-3 minutes until thick and creamy.

Consume immediately.

READY IN
10
MINUTES

PER SERVING:
166 Calories
14g Carbs
23g Protein
2g Fat

Creamy coconut cheesecake

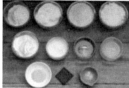

MIKAYLA FIT

for the base:
⅔ cup ground almonds

½ cup unsweetened coconut flakes, finely ground

3 Tbsps. melted coconut oil

2 tsps. maple syrup

1 tsp. vanilla extract

¼ tsp. sea salt

for the cheesecake layer:
⅓ cup unsweetened coconut flakes, finely ground

1 cup cream cheese at room temperature (use dairy free if preferred)

⅔ cup Greek yogurt (use dairy free if preferred)

⅓ cup vanilla or coconut flavor whey or rice protein powder

1 tsp. vanilla extract

a small pinch of sea salt

2 fl oz. unsweetened coconut milk (long life drink)

for the topping:
2 squares dark chocolate, grated

SERVES 8

PER SERVING:
279 Calories
7g Carbs
11g Protein
23g Fat

Preheat oven to 170°C/ 350°F. Line the base of a medium-sized loaf pan with baking paper.

Place all of the base ingredients in a large bowl. Stir until thoroughly combined. Transfer to the pan and press down firmly. Bake for 10-15 minutes, or until golden brown. Allow to cool completely.

Meanwhile, place the cheesecake layer ingredients in a bowl. Stir until thoroughly combined. Pour the mixture over the cooled base and spread evenly.

Freeze for 1 hour or until firm enough to remove from tin. Transfer to a chopping board and cut into 8 pieces. Serve topped with grated dark chocolate.

Store any leftovers in an airtight container and refrigerate for up to 4 days or freeze on same day.

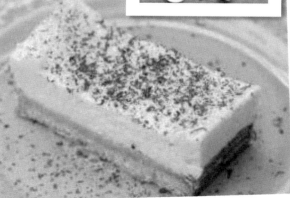

Indulgent cookie cakes

MIKAYLA FIT

5¼ fl oz. unsweetened coconut milk

2 Tbsps. flaxseed, ground

2 Tbsps. ground almonds

3 Tbsps. coconut flour

1⅓ cups gluten-free flour of choice

2 Tbsps. organic cocoa powder

1 tsp. baking soda

4 Tbsps. chocolate flavor whey or rice protein powder (optional)

6 pitted dates, chopped finely

3 heaping Tbsps. dark chocolate (minimum 70% cocoa), cut into small pieces

3 Tbsps. coconut oil, melted

1¾ fl oz. olive oil

3 Tbsps. stevia (or natural sweetener of your choice) plus a bit extra for topping

2 tsps. vanilla extract

MAKES 12 COOKIES

PER COOKIE:
238 Calories
17g Carbs
10g Protein
14g Fat

Preheat oven to 180°C/350°F.

Mix the coconut milk, flaxseed and almonds in a bowl.

Mix the flours, cocoa powder, baking soda, protein powder, dates and chocolate in a bowl. Add the oils, stevia and vanilla extract to the coconut milk mixture. Stir well. Leave to stand for 10 minutes.

Pour the wet mixture into the dry mixture and stir well. Add a drop of water if needed. The consistency should be of a thick paste.

Line several trays with baking paper. Roll small amounts of the mixture into balls. Press gently into disc shapes (maximum 15mm thick) onto the baking paper. Allow some space between the cookies, as they will spread whilst baking. Sprinkle a little extra stevia on top of each cookie, and gently press it into the dough. Bake for 7 minutes. Transfer to a wire rack to cool.

Store in an airtight container at room temperature for up to 3 days.

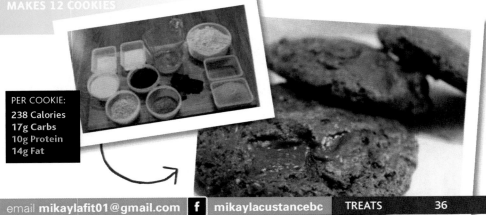

Grab & go protein snack

READY IN 5 MINUTES

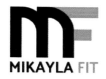

⅘ cup cottage cheese (use dairy free if preferred)
1 kiwi, diced
1 Tbsp. flaked almonds
2 tsps. mixed seeds (e.g. flaxseed, sesame seeds, sunflower seeds)

Put the cottage cheese in a bowl and top with the kiwi, almonds and seeds.

Store in an airtight container and refrigerate for up to 2 days.

SERVES 1

PER SERVING:
339 Calories
23g Carbs
28g Protein
15g Fat

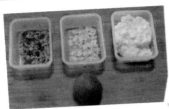
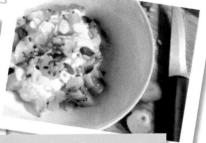

Buttery scallion scrambled eggs

READY IN 10 MINUTES

4 eggs
1 egg white
a pinch of salt and pepper
1 heaping tsp. butter
2 scallions, finely chopped

Crack the eggs into a jug. Add the egg white, season with salt and pepper and whisk well with a fork.

Melt the butter in a pan and add the scallions. Add the eggs to the pan and stir until the eggs are cooked. Serve.

Consume immediately.

Serving suggestion:

Serve with steamed greens of your choice.

SERVES 1

PER SERVING:
357 Calories
3g Carbs
30g Protein
25g Fat

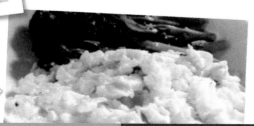

Spiced apple power porridge

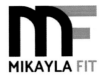

½ cup porridge oats, (use gluten free oats if preferred)
3.5 fl oz. cold water (or use milk of your choice)
1 medium sized apple, diced
1 Tbsp. flaxseed, ground
1 tsp. ground cinnamon

SERVES 1

Place the oats and water in a saucepan. Stir and cook over a medium heat for 3-4 minutes, stirring continuously.

If the mixture is a little dry, add a splash more water or milk.

When the porridge starts to thicken, add the diced apple and cook for 2-3 minutes. Stir in the flaxseed.

Spoon the contents into a bowl, and sprinkle with cinnamon.

Consume immediately.

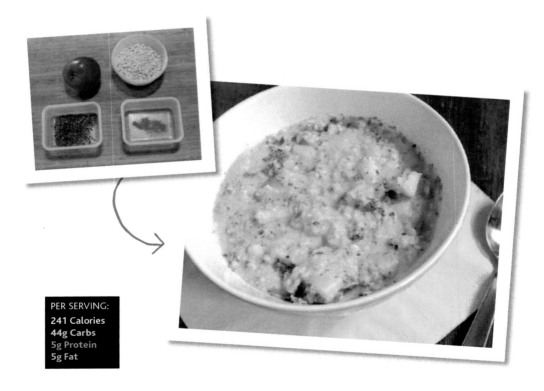

PER SERVING:
241 Calories
44g Carbs
5g Protein
5g Fat

Bacon & egg frittata

MIKAYLA FIT

3 medium sized eggs
5-6 cherry tomatoes, halved
1 tsp. organic butter or coconut oil
2 slices unsmoked back bacon, diced (use vegetarian bacon if preferred*)
sprinkle fresh chopped parsley

SERVES 1

Note: Some meat free alternatives contain gluten and/or MSG. Please check the label before you buy!

Preheat oven to 175°C/350°F.

Beat the eggs in a bowl until stiff peaks form.

Gently melt the butter / oil in a skillet or frying pan and fry the bacon until crispy. Add the tomatoes and cook for 2 minutes.

Pour the egg batter into the skillet so that it covers the base of the pan evenly. Cook on a medium heat for two minutes, then bake in the oven for 15 minutes.

Remove the frittata gently from the skillet, loosening with a spatula. Serve garnished with a fresh salad.

Store in an airtight container and refrigerate for up to 24 hours.

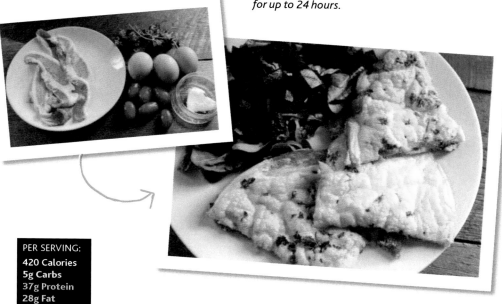

PER SERVING:
420 Calories
5g Carbs
37g Protein
28g Fat

Breakfast burrito

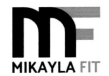

3 medium sized eggs, yolks and whites separated
1 tsp. coconut oil or butter
½ a small red onion, finely chopped
1 tomato, finely chopped
1 green chilli, finely chopped
½ a bell-pepper (any color), diced
handful fresh cilantro, finely chopped
5¾ oz. cooked chicken, sliced
½ a small avocado, cut into small chunks

SERVES 1

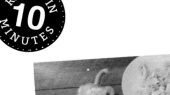

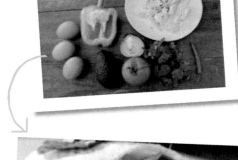

Whisk the egg whites for one minute.

Melt half of the oil or butter over a medium heat in a skillet or frying pan. Pour the egg whites into the pan, tilting the base of the pan to spread them evenly.

Cook for around 1-2 minutes until the egg is cooked through. Use a spatula to gently loosen and slide onto a plate.

Sauté the onion with the remaining oil for one minute then add the tomato, chilli, bell-pepper, cilantro and chicken.

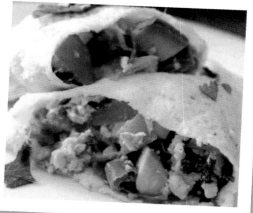

PER SERVING:
540 Calories
20g Carbs
43g Protein
32g Fat

Whisk egg yolks and pour into the pan, mixing well into the other ingredients. Season with salt and pepper.

When the egg yolks are cooked, add the avocado then spoon the mixture onto the egg white. Roll the egg white up into a burrito.

Consume immediately.

Summer fruit pancakes

MIKAYLA FIT

3 tsps. coconut flour
2 medium sized eggs
1 egg yolk
½ tsp. ground cinnamon
2 tsps. stevia (or natural
sweetener of your choice)
3 tsps. coconut oil
1 Tbsp. plain or Greek yogurt (use
dairy free yogurt if preferred)
1 cup mixed berries

SERVES 2

Suggestion:
Berries are medium / low sugar fruits, ideal if you are watching your carb intake

Place the flour, eggs, cinnamon and stevia in a blender and mix until smooth. Add a bit more flour if the mixture is too thin, or if the mixture is too thick, add a drop of cold water or unsweetened almond milk. The aim is to achieve a pourable but not runny consistency.

Heat the coconut oil in a pan over a medium/high heat and then pour in around 1¾ fl oz. of the mixture into the center of the pan.

Move the pan around gently to even out the mixture into a circular shape. When small holes appear in the pancake (around 1-2 minutes), turn it over and cook for 1-2 minutes, until golden. Transfer to a plate.

Repeat with the remaining batter. Serve with yogurt and berries.

Store any leftover pancakes in an airtight container and refrigerate for up to 4 days.

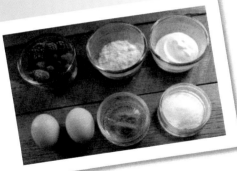

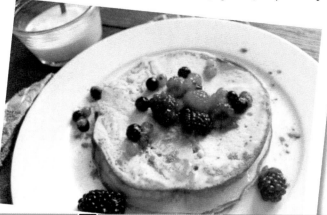

PER SERVING:
220 Calories
9g Carbs
10g Protein
16g Fat

Fruit & nut porridge

MIKAYLA FIT

⅔ cup porridge oats, (use gluten free oats if preferred)
3.5 fl oz. cold water (or use milk of your choice)
1 tsp. stevia (or natural sweetener of your choice)
1 kiwi, diced
1 tsp. flaked almonds
5 dried pitted prunes, chopped

SERVES 1

Place the oats and water in a saucepan. Stir and cook over a medium heat for 3-4 minutes, stirring continuously.

If the mixture is a little dry, add a splash more water or milk.

Remove pan from the heat and stir in the stevia.

Spoon the contents into a bowl. Add the kiwi, almonds, and prunes.

Consume immediately.

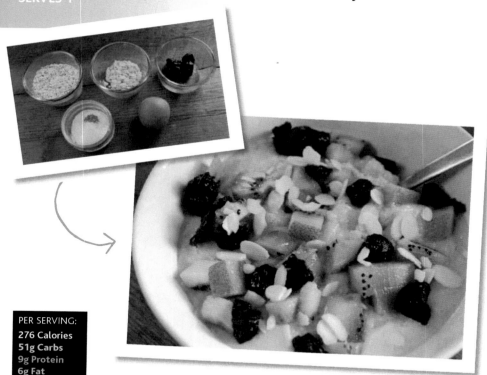

PER SERVING:
276 Calories
51g Carbs
9g Protein
6g Fat

Buttery eggs

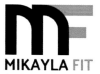
2 medium sized eggs
2 organic oatcakes (use gluten free oatcakes if preferred)
1 tsp. organic butter or olive oil
salt and pepper
handful spinach leaves, chopped
5 cherry tomatoes, halved

SERVES 1

Boil the eggs in a pan of salted water for 10 minutes. While the eggs are cooking, steam the chopped spinach leaves gently for 4-5 minutes.

Cover the eggs in cold water for one minute to cool, then peel. Place the eggs in a bowl and add the butter / oil. Season with salt and pepper and mash thoroughly with a fork.

Spread thickly onto the oatcakes. Serve with the spinach and tomatoes.

Consume immediately.

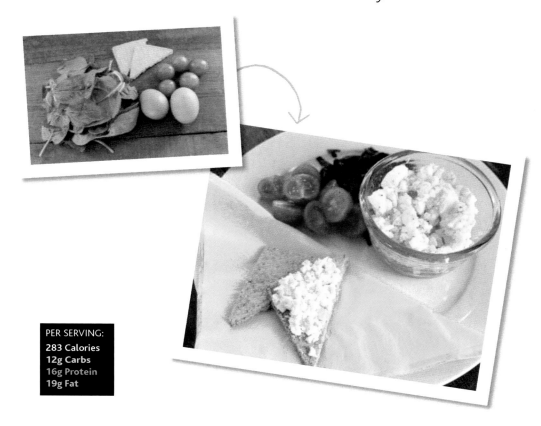

PER SERVING:
283 Calories
12g Carbs
16g Protein
19g Fat

Indian spiced muffins

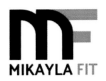

MIKAYLA FIT

1 tsp. ghee or coconut oil plus extra to grease tin
1 tsp. curry powder
1 small red onion, finely chopped
1 red chili pepper, finely chopped
6 eggs
½ tsp. cumin seeds
a pinch of sea salt
a pinch of ground black pepper
a handful of spinach, finely chopped
2 Tbsps. peas

MAKES 8 MUFFINS

Preheat oven to 180°C/350°F. Grease 8 compartments of a muffin tin.

Melt the ghee / oil in a saucepan over a medium heat. Add the onion, chili pepper and curry powder, stir well and sauté for 4 minutes, stirring occasionally.

Remove pan from heat and transfer the mixture to a plate to cool for 5 minutes.

Meanwhile place the eggs, cumin, salt and pepper in a large jug and whisk well. Add the peas and spinach and stir.

Stir in the onion mixture.

Pour the mixture into the compartments. Bake for 15 minutes or until firm.

Store any leftovers in an airtight container and refrigerate for up to 2 days.

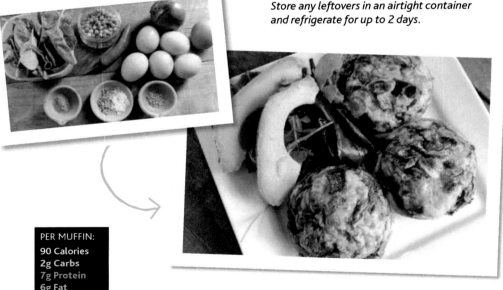

PER MUFFIN:
90 Calories
2g Carbs
7g Protein
6g Fat

Piled-high protein breakfast

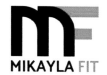

MIKAYLA FIT

2 medium sized eggs
3½ cups fresh spinach
1 Tbsp. plain cashews
8 plum tomatoes, halved
¼ bell-pepper (any color), diced
1 tsp. olive oil mixed with 1 tsp. balsamic vinegar

SERVES 1

Boil the eggs in a saucepan of water for 8 minutes.

Meanwhile, steam the spinach gently for 3-4 minutes until wilted.

Remove the eggs from the saucepan, and immerse in cold water for 2 minutes, to cool. Peel and slice the eggs.

Place the spinach in a serving bowl and drizzle over the oil / vinegar. Add the eggs, bell-pepper, tomatoes and cashew nuts.

Consume immediately.

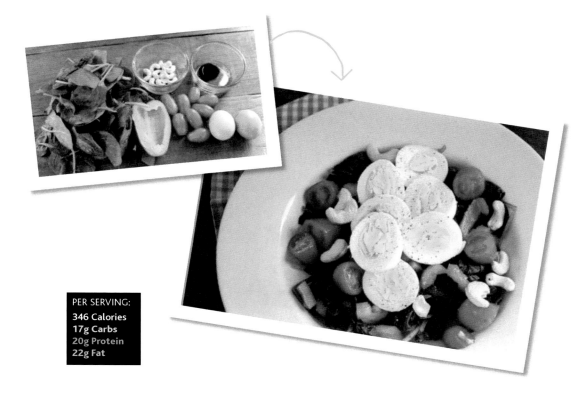

PER SERVING:
346 Calories
17g Carbs
20g Protein
22g Fat

Breakfast protein oat bars

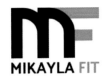

MIKAYLA FIT

½ cup oats (use gluten free if preferred)

½ cup chocolate flavor whey or rice protein powder (optional)

1 Tbsp. cocoa powder

2 Tbsps. dried dates, chopped and pre-soaked in cold water for 30 minutes

2 Tbsps. cashews, chopped

1 Tbsp. unsweetened coconut flakes

1 tsp. vanilla extract

¼ tsp. sea salt

3.4 fl oz. cold water or unsweetened almond milk

2 tsps. almond butter

MAKES 8 BARS

Place all of the ingredients in a bowl and mix well to combine thoroughly.

Line the base of a 6x6 inch tin with greaseproof paper.

Pour the mixture into the tin and press down firmly to cover the base of the tin.

Refrigerate for one hour or more. Cut into 8 pieces.

Store any leftovers in an airtight container and refrigerate for up to 3 days.

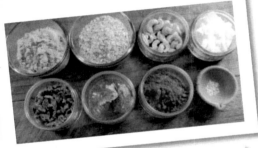

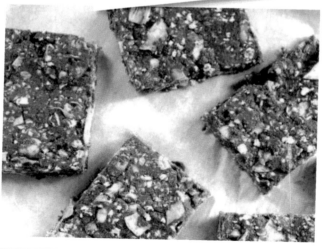

PER BAR:
122 Calories
9g Carbs
8g Protein
6g Fat

Tasty veg pizza

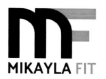

small amount of coconut oil for greasing
4 medium sized eggs
3 egg whites
Himalayan pink salt to season
⅔ cup porridge oats (use gluten free oats if preferred)
7 cherry tomatoes, halved
2 cups baby leaf spinach, finely chopped
1 green chili pepper, finely chopped
½ a large green bell-pepper, finely chopped
1 tsp. paprika
½ tsp. dried oregano
⅓ cup low fat hard cheese, grated (use a dairy free cheese if preferred)

MAKES 8 SLICES

Top tip:
This pizza makes a great portable snack. Tastes great hot or cold

Preheat oven to 150°C/300°F.

Lightly grease a large round ovenproof dish with coconut oil or butter.

Whisk the eggs and egg whites in a jug and season well with Himalayan salt. Add the oats, vegetables, dried spices and herbs. Stir well. Pour into the dish and cook for 10 minutes.

Remove from oven and sprinkle on the cheese. Cook for a further 5 minutes, or until center of pizza is cooked.

Store any leftovers in an airtight container and refrigerate for up to 2 days.

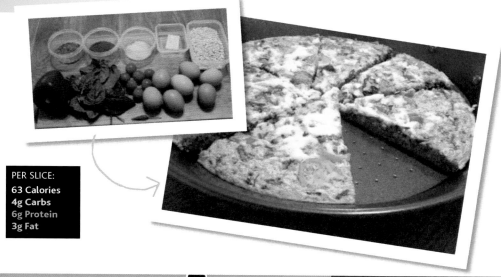

PER SLICE:
63 Calories
4g Carbs
6g Protein
3g Fat

Poached salmon protein brunch

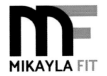

MIKAYLA FIT

3.5 oz. salmon fillet
1 handful kale
¼ cup closed cup mushrooms
1 tsp. organic butter or coconut oil
2 medium sized eggs
salt and pepper to season

READY IN 10 MINUTES

SERVES 1

In a large shallow pan, bring some water to the boil - just a couple of inches of water is adequate for shallow poaching.

Add the salmon and poach gently for 8 minutes, turning on each side as it cooks.

In a separate saucepan, melt the butter over a medium heat and cook the mushrooms for 3-4 minutes until soft.

Bring a small pan of water to the boil (again just a couple of inches of water). Reduce the heat to a very gentle simmer and carefully add the eggs.

Poach for 2-4 minutes (2 minutes is ideal for a runny egg).

Add the kale to the saucepan with the salmon and cook it in the water for several minutes. Top up with water if necessary.

When the salmon is cooked - it should be a light pink color throughout - remove it from the saucepan and set aside. Drain the kale and leave for a few minutes to remove excess water.

Place the kale and the mushrooms on a plate and top with the salmon and the eggs. Season well with salt and pepper.

Consume immediately.

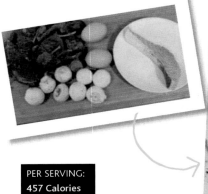

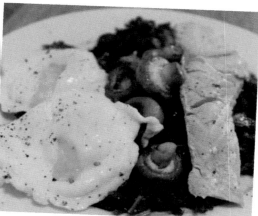

PER SERVING:
457 Calories
6g Carbs
42g Protein
30g Fat

Summer fruit porridge

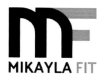

MIKAYLA FIT

½ cup porridge oats (use gluten free oats if preferred)
5 fl oz. cold water
⅓ cup mixed berries (fresh or frozen) plus a few extra for topping
3 Tbsps. strawberry or vanilla flavor whey or rice protein powder (optional)

SERVES 1

Top tip:

This high carb recipe makes an ideal post-workout breakfast.

If possible, presoak the oats for 8 hours or more. Soaking the oats for 10-12 hours overnight makes it easier for the body to digest. It also speeds up the cooking process, which is ideal if you are short on time in the mornings

Mix the oats and water in a saucepan over a medium heat. Bring to the boil then reduce to a gentle simmer. Stir constantly until the porridge starts to thicken.

Add the berries and continue to cook, stirring for 1-2 minutes. Add more water if required if the mixture looks too thick.

Taste test the porridge to ensure that the fruit is heated through. Remove from heat and stir in the protein powder until thoroughly combined. Sprinkle over a few extra berries and serve.

Consume immediately.

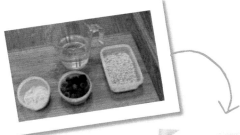

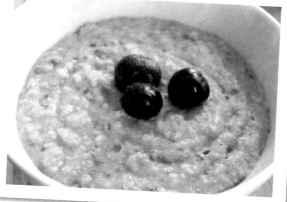

PER SERVING:
346 Calories
36g Carbs
37g Protein
6g Fat

Banana protein pancakes

MIKAYLA FIT

4 medium sized eggs
1 egg white
¼ cup vanilla or chocolate flavor whey or rice protein powder
1 medium sized banana
⅖ cup whole porridge oats (use gluten free oats if preferred)
1 tsp. cinnamon
2 tsps. stevia or honey
1 Tbsp. coconut flour
1 Tbsp. coconut oil

MAKES 4 PANCAKES

Put all of the ingredients except for the oil into a blender and mix together. Add a little water if necessary to achieve the right consistency. The mixture should be quite thick but pourable.

Heat a small amount of the oil in a large non stick pan, over a medium / high heat.

Pour a quarter of the mixture into the center of the pan. Move the pan around gently to even out the mixture into a circular shape.

When small holes appear in the pancake, turn (or flip) it over and heat on the other side for 1-2 minutes. Transfer to a plate.

Add more oil and repeat with the remaining batter.

Store any leftover pancakes in an airtight container and refrigerate for up to 3 days.

PER PANCAKE:
193 Calories
14g Carbs
14g Protein
9g Fat

Prune & sweet potato pancakes

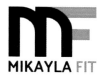

MIKAYLA FIT

For the pancakes:

1 cup sweet potato, peeled and diced

5 medium sized eggs

2 Tbsps. chocolate flavor whey or rice protein powder (optional)

half a medium sized banana

1 tsp. ground cinnamon

1 tsp. stevia or honey

1 Tbsp. coconut flour

2 Tbsps. pitted prunes, chopped roughly

2 Tbsps. coconut oil

For the blueberry sauce:

½ cup blueberries

juice of half a lemon

1 tsp. stevia (or natural sweetener of your choice)

MAKES 9 SERVINGS

Bring a saucepan of water to the boil. Add the sweet potato and simmer for around 8 minutes until soft. Remove from heat, drain and leave to cool.

Mash the sweet potato gently in a fine sieve to remove excess water.

Put all of the other pancake ingredients (except for the coconut oil) into a blender and pulse until smooth. Allow to stand for 10 minutes.

RECIPE CONTINUED ON NEXT PAGE >>

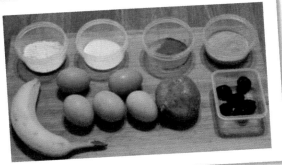

PER SERVING:
114 Calories
9g Carbs
6g Protein
6g Fat

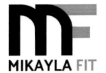

Heat a small amount of the coconut oil in a non stick pan, over a medium / high heat. Pour a small amount of the pancake mixture into the center of the pan (6 inch diameter).

Move the pan around gently to even out the mixture into a circular shape. When small holes appear in the pancake, turn or flip it over and cook for 1-2 minutes.

Transfer pancake to a plate. Add more oil and repeat the process with remaining batter.

Mix the blueberries with a splash of cold water and warm in a saucepan over a gentle heat. Add the lemon juice and stevia and stir. Cook for 3-4 minutes then leave to cool for several minutes.

Store any leftover pancakes in an airtight container and refrigerate for up to 2 days.

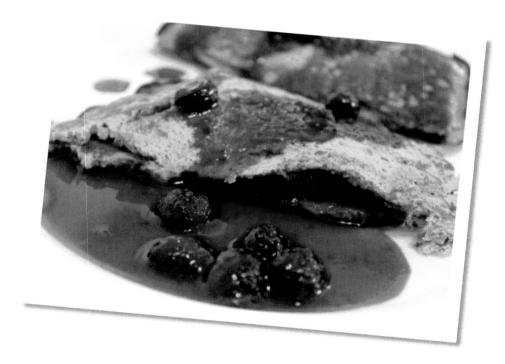

Citrus protein yogurt breakfast bowls

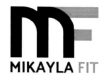

MIKAYLA FIT

2 fl oz. + 1 fl oz. recently boiled water

¾ tsp. vanilla extract or vanilla bean paste

2 strips of lemon rind

1 tsp. stevia (or use natural sweetener of your choice)

1 navel orange, peeled and sliced

¼ cup raspberries

1 tsp. chia seeds

2 tsps. lemon juice

1¼ cups Greek yogurt (use dairy free if preferred)

¼ cup vanilla flavor whey or rice protein powder (optional)

SERVES 2

Pour 2 fl oz. recently boiled water into a small saucepan and add the lemon rind, vanilla extract and stevia. Simmer gently for 6 minutes then remove from heat. Remove lemon rind and leave to cool.

Add the orange slices and stir.

In a separate saucepan mash the raspberries. Add the chia seeds, lemon juice and 1 fl oz. recently boiled water. Stir well and cook over a medium / low heat for 4 minutes, stirring occasionally. Remove from heat.

Mix the protein powder (if using) with the yogurt. Spoon the yogurt into two small serving bowls. Add a layer of raspberry chia jam. Top with the orange slices in the juice. Add a drizzle of raspberry chia jam. Serve.

Refrigerate any leftovers for up to 2 days.

PER SERVING:
260 Calories
22g Carbs
25g Protein
8g Fat

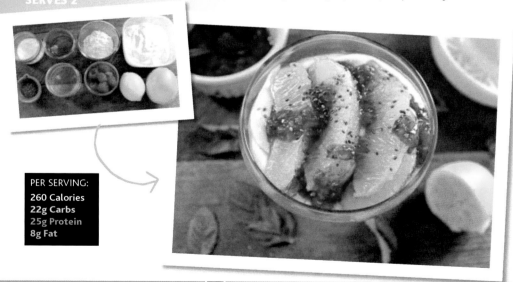

Meat & nuts

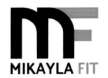

MIKAYLA FIT

1 tsp. coconut oil
5¼ oz. lean stir fry beef strips
½ tsp. paprika
½ tsp. sea salt flakes
½ tsp. black pepper
handful fresh spinach
¼ cup walnuts

SERVES 1

READY IN
10
MINUTES

Heat the oil in a frying pan or skillet over a medium heat.

Add the spices and stir for 10 seconds.

Add the beef and cook for 2-3 minutes, stirring.

Add the spinach and cook, stirring until wilted.

Transfer the contents of the pan in to a bowl and sprinkle over the walnuts.

Consume immediately.

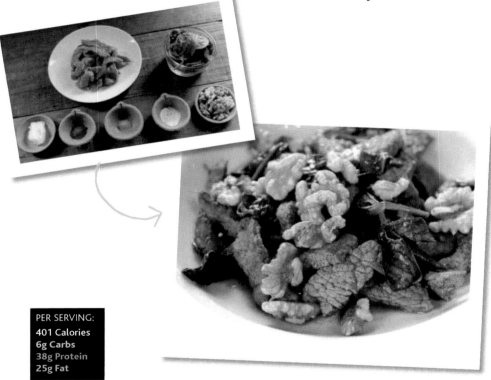

PER SERVING:
401 Calories
6g Carbs
38g Protein
25g Fat

Mexican butterfly chicken breast

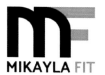

MIKAYLA FIT

2 x 7 oz. fresh chicken breasts
1 Tbsp. extra virgin olive oil
1 tsp. paprika
½ tsp. chili powder
½ tsp. ground cilantro
⅓ tsp. cumin seeds
a pinch of salt and black pepper
1 red bell-pepper, sliced
1 green bell-pepper, sliced
2 small red onions, sliced
14 cherry tomatoes, halved
2 lime wedges to serve

SERVES 2

Place the chicken breasts between two layers of cling film. Hit the chicken breasts with a rolling pin to tenderise the meat.

Drizzle the olive oil over the chicken breasts. Sprinkle the paprika, chilli powder, cilantro powder, cumin seeds and salt and pepper evenly over the chicken.

Cover with cling film and refrigerate for at least half an hour, but longer will provide a better flavor.

Preheat oven to 180°C/350°F. Place the chicken breasts, peppers, onions and tomatoes on a baking tray. Cook for 20-25 minutes, ensuring the chicken is cooked thoroughly. Serve with lime wedges

Store any leftovers in an airtight container and refrigerate for up to 2 days.

Place a chicken breast on a chopping board. Place your hand flat on top of it and, using a sharp knife, slice into one side of the breast, starting at the thicker end and ending at the thin point. Be careful not to cut all the way through to the other side. Open out the breast so that it resembles a butterfly. Repeat with the other chicken breast.

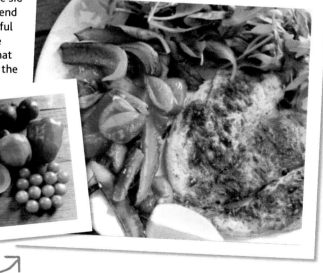

PER SERVING:
350 Calories
18g Carbs
47g Protein
10g Fat

Pan-fried chili & lemon haddock

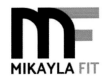

MIKAYLA FIT

¾ tsp. paprika
½ tsp. dried red chili flakes
a pinch of salt and pepper
2 x 5 oz. haddock fillets
juice of ½ a lemon
2 tsps. butter or coconut oil

SERVES 2

Sprinkle the paprika, chili flakes, salt, pepper and lemon juice over the haddock.

Melt the butter/ oil in a frying pan over a medium heat.

Place the haddock in the pan, skin side down and fry gently for around 8 minutes or until cooked throughout. Serve.

Consume immediately.

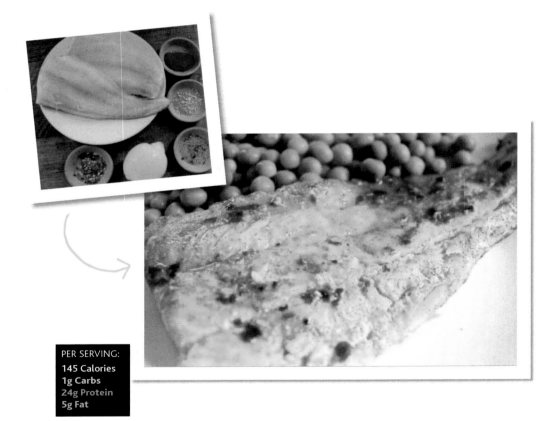

PER SERVING:
145 Calories
1g Carbs
24g Protein
5g Fat

O-mega salad

1 medium sized egg
3 small new potatoes, chopped into small pieces
1 tsp. organic butter or coconut oil
4½ oz. fresh chicken breast/ vegetarian chicken*, cut into strips
½ tsp. dried oregano
few handfuls of mixed lettuce, torn into small pieces
¼ red bell-pepper, diced
¼ yellow bell-pepper, diced
4 cherry tomatoes, chopped
small handful samphire
⅙ cup cucumber, sliced
1½ tsps. organic olive oil
2 tsps. omega sprinkle (e.g flaxseed, sesame seeds, sunflower seeds)
salt and pepper to season

SERVES 1

Bring a saucepan of water to the boil and cook the egg for around 10 minutes. Remove from water and set aside.

Add the potatoes to the water and simmer for 10 minutes or until soft. Remove from the water and drain.

Melt the butter or oil over a medium heat in a frying pan and add the chicken. Sprinkle over the oregano, and cook for around 8 minutes, turning occasionally to brown on all sides. Once cooked, remove chicken from pan and set aside.

In a salad bowl, mix together the lettuce, bell-peppers, tomatoes, samphire and cucumber. Pour over the olive oil and mix well.

Slice the egg into quarters and arrange over the salad leaves, along with the chicken. Top with the omega sprinkle and season with salt and pepper.

Store in an airtight container and refrigerate for up to 24 hours.

Note: Some meat free alternatives contain gluten and/or MSG. Please check the label before you buy!

PER SERVING:
482 Calories
19g Carbs
52g Protein
22g Fat

Egg drop soup

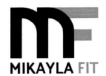

17½ fl oz. fresh stock
(see recipes on right)
7 oz. fresh chicken breast,
diced
2 cups frozen vegetables (broccoli,
carrots, sweetcorn, beans, etc)
2 medium sized eggs, beaten
3 scallions, finely sliced
salt and pepper

READY IN 10 MINUTES

SERVES 2

In a large saucepan, bring the stock to a gentle simmer. Add the chicken and vegetables. Simmer rapidly for 5 minutes.

Pour eggs into the soup in a steady stream, then stir gently while the egg cooks. Season with salt and pepper to taste. Spoon into bowls and garnish with scallions.

Consume immediately.

Home-made chicken stock: Chicken stock is quick to make and so good for you! Place a whole chicken carcass in a large pan full of water (enough to cover the chicken). Season well with salt and pepper and add a bay leaf.

Simmer for 2 hours. Remove from heat and allow to cool completely, then drain the liquid from the carcass. Discard carcass and bay leaf. The stock can be frozen or kept in the fridge for several days

Home-made vegetable stock: Add a drop of olive oil to a large saucepan over a medium heat. Add a large diced white onion, a sliced leek, and chopped carrot and sweat for 2-3 minutes. Add enough cold water to cover the vegetables and turn up the heat to high. Add some finely chopped garlic, one stick of chopped celery, several chopped tomatoes, 1 tsp. dried parsley, half a tsp. of black pepper, half a tsp. salt, 1 tsp. dried fennel, a sprig of fresh or 1 tsp. dried rosemary.

Stir well, bring to the boil, cover, then reduce to a simmer for 25 minutes. Pour the stock through a sieve. Discard the vegetable pieces or re-use. The liquid stock can be stored in the fridge for up to three days or frozen in batches for future use.

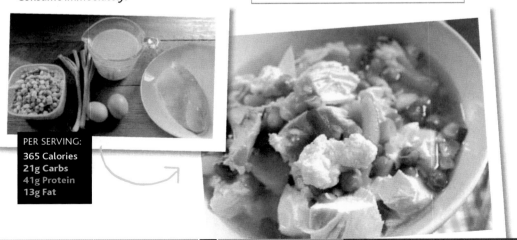

PER SERVING:
365 Calories
21g Carbs
41g Protein
13g Fat

Thai chicken noodle soup

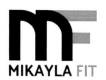

1 tsp. ghee or coconut oil

1 large stick lemongrass, minced

1 inch piece fresh galangal or ginger, peeled and finely chopped

4 small shallots, finely chopped

2-3 green chili peppers, finely chopped

2 cloves fresh garlic, finely chopped

4 scallions, finely chopped

28.75 fl oz. chicken stock or recently boiled water

juice of one lime

a pinch of sea salt

a pinch of ground black pepper

1 Tbsp. fish sauce (nam pla)

10 oz. stir fry vegetables

35.25 oz. skinless chicken drumsticks

4 fl oz. unsweetened coconut milk

⅔ cup (per person) rice vermicelli noodles

SERVES 5

Melt the ghee / oil in a large saucepan over a medium heat. Add the lemongrass, galangal, shallots and chili peppers and sauté for 2-3 minutes.

Add the garlic and scallions and cook for 1-2 minutes, stirring frequently. Add the chicken stock and bring to the boil, then reduce heat to simmer gently.

Add the lime juice, salt and pepper, fish sauce, stir fry vegetables and chicken. Cover and cook for 20 minutes or until the chicken is thoroughly cooked.

Meanwhile, bring a saucepan of water to the boil. Add the rice noodles and cook for 2-3 minutes, until cooked. Drain well and leave to stand for several minutes, then stir into the soup.

Add the coconut milk to the soup, stir and cook for one minute. Serve.

Store any leftovers in an airtight container and refrigerate for up to 3 days or freeze on same day.

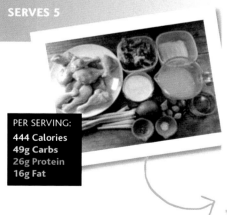

PER SERVING:
444 Calories
49g Carbs
26g Protein
16g Fat

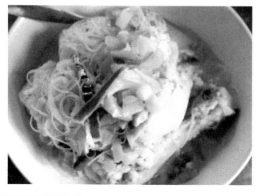

Italian inspired stuffed peppers

2 large bell-peppers (any colour)
½ tsp. butter or cooking fat of your choice
1 small onion, finely diced
1 cup mushrooms, roughly chopped
1 heaping Tbsp. tomato purée
½ tsp. dried Italian herbs
a pinch of salt and pepper
4 eggs
2 Tbsps. grated Cheddar or similar hard cheese (use dairy free if preferred)

SERVES 2

Preheat the oven to 200°C/400°F.

Cut the peppers down the middle (lengthwise). Remove the pith and seeds and discard. Place the peppers (skin side down) in an ovenproof dish.

Melt the butter in a frying pan over a medium heat. Add the onion and mushrooms. Fry gently for 5 minutes, stirring regularly.

Add the tomato purée, salt, pepper and Italian herbs. Cook for 2 minutes, stirring. Spoon the mixture into each of the pepper halves.

Make a small well in the mixture. Carefully crack one egg into each well, ensuring that the egg doesn't overrun.

Sprinkle the cheese over the egg. Bake for 20 minutes.

Consume immediately.

PER SERVING:
322 Calories
19g Carbs
21g Protein
18g Fat

Cauliflower chicken

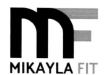

MIKAYLA FIT

1 large cauliflower head, grated
1 Tbsp. organic butter or coconut oil
21¼ oz. fresh chicken breast/meat free chicken*, cut into strips
1 medium sized white onion, finely chopped
2 garlic cloves, finely chopped
1 green bell-pepper, diced
1 x 400g can tomatoes
10½ fl oz. chicken/vegetable stock (see recipes on page 58)
1 tsp. ground cumin
1 tsp. sea salt flakes
⅔ cup frozen peas

SERVES 4

Grate the cauliflower or blend in a food processor.

In a large saucepan, melt the butter or oil over a medium / high heat and add the chicken. Cook for 4-6 minutes until browned all over.

Add the onion, garlic and bell-pepper and sauté for 2-3 minutes.

Add the tomatoes, stock, cumin, salt and cauliflower. Stir well. Simmer covered for 10 minutes.

Add the peas and simmer for 2-3 minutes then serve.

Once cooled, store any leftovers in an airtight container and refrigerate for up to 3 days or freeze on same day.

* **Note:** *Some meat free alternatives contain gluten and/or MSG. Please check the label before you buy!*

PER SERVING:
320 Calories
17g Carbs
45g Protein
8g Fat

King prawn risotto with peas & fennel

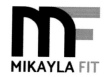

MIKAYLA FIT

2 tsps. butter or coconut oil
1 medium brown onion, finely diced
2 garlic cloves, finely diced
1 tsp. fennel seeds
1 cup arborio rice
15 fl oz. hot vegetable stock (made with one organic stock cube)
½ cup frozen peas
10.5 oz. raw peeled king prawns
grated zest of ½ a lemon
a squeeze of lemon juice
a small handful of fresh chives, finely chopped
a pinch of sea salt
a pinch of black pepper

SERVES 3

Melt the butter / oil in a large saucepan over a medium heat. Add the onion, garlic and fennel seeds. Cook gently for 5 minutes, stirring frequently.

Add the rice and stock to the saucepan and stir. Cover and simmer gently for 10 minutes, stirring occasionally. Add a little boiling water if the mixture is too dry. Cook for a further 10 minutes, stirring occasionally.

Add the peas and cook for 5 minutes.

Add the prawns, stir well and cover. Cook for 5 minutes, or until the prawns are cooked throughout.

Add the lemon zest, lemon juice, chives and salt and pepper.

Store any leftovers in an airtight container and refrigerate for up to 3 days or freeze on same day.

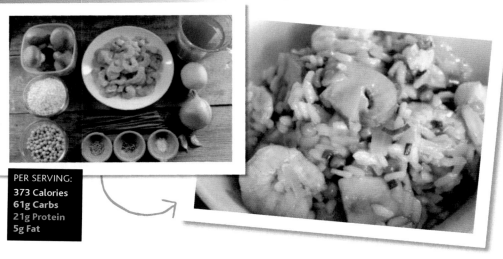

PER SERVING:
373 Calories
61g Carbs
21g Protein
5g Fat

Sesame chicken

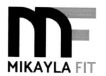

MIKAYLA FIT

1 Tbsp. coconut oil, melted
6¼ oz. chicken breast/meat free
chicken*, cut into strips
salt and pepper
1½ tsps. tahini
1½ tsps. sherry vinegar
½ tsp. olive oil
1 small carrot, grated
5 radishes, sliced
large handful mixed lettuce leaves
sprinkle of sesame seeds to garnish

SERVES 1

** **Note:** Some meat free alternatives contain gluten and/or MSG. Please check the label before you buy!*

Season the chicken with salt and pepper and mix with half of the oil. In a skillet, melt the remaining oil over a medium/high heat.

Cook the chicken for 10 minutes, turning halfway. Remove from heat and set aside.

In a jug, combine the tahini, sherry vinegar and olive oil.

In a bowl, mix the chicken with carrots, radish and lettuce. Drizzle the tahini dressing on top and mix well. Top with the cooked chicken and garnish with sesame seeds.

Store any leftovers in an airtight container and refrigerate for up to 24 hours.

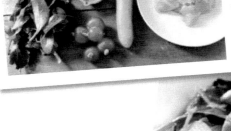

PER SERVING:
446 Calories
11g Carbs
42g Protein
26g Fat

Chicken meatballs

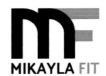

12.25oz. fresh chicken breast/
vegetarian chicken*, diced
1 large carrot, grated
2 garlic cloves, finely chopped
1 cup fresh coconut, grated
1 medium sized egg
2 tsps. curry powder
½ tsp. sea salt flakes
handful parsley or cilantro
2 tsps. coconut oil
wedges of lemon to serve
plain yogurt to serve (use
dairy free yoghurt if preferred)

MAKES 20 MEATBALLS

Note: Some meat free alternatives contain gluten and/or MSG. Please check the label before you buy!

Put everything except for the coconut oil into a food processor and blend into a smooth paste. Using your hands, form the mixture into 20 meatballs.

In a large pan, melt the coconut oil over a high heat. When the oil is hot, put the meatballs in the pan and cook for 2 minutes. Reduce the heat to medium. Roll each meatball over and cook for a further 5 minutes.

Serve with lemon wedges and a plain yogurt dip.

Store any leftovers in an airtight container and refrigerate for up to 3 days.

Suggestion:

These are an ideal portable snack or as a meal served with a healthy accompaniment e.g. a salad and sweet potato.

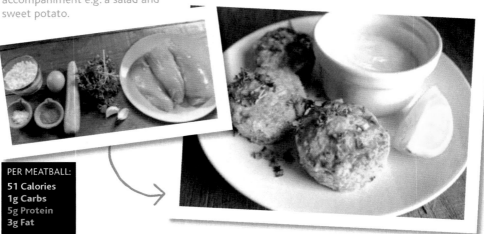

PER MEATBALL:
51 Calories
1g Carbs
5g Protein
3g Fat

Pork & apple meatballs

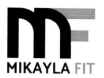

MIKAYLA FIT

2 tsps. coconut oil

for the meatballs:

17.5 oz. lean pork mince
1 small apple, grated
1 tsp. dried sage or rosemary
1 egg
a pinch of sea salt
a pinch of ground black pepper
2 scallions, finely chopped

MAKES 11 MEATBALLS

Place the ingredients in a large bowl and mix well with your hands, until thoroughly combined. Use your hands to mash the mixture together.

Roll the mixture into 11 compact balls.

Heat half of the coconut oil in a frying pan over a medium/low heat. Add 5-6 of the balls and fry gently for 5 minutes, turning occasionally, until cooked in the center.

Remove from the pan and transfer to a plate.

Repeat steps with the remaining oil and meatballs. Serve.

Store any leftovers in an airtight container and refrigerate for up to 2 days or freeze on same day.

Serving suggestion:

Serve with rice (optional) and salad, or enjoy as a snack.

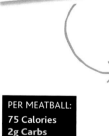

PER MEATBALL:
75 Calories
2g Carbs
10g Protein
3g Fat

Lentil pepper soup

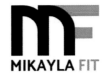
MIKAYLA FIT

1⅓ cups red lentils
34¼ fl oz. fresh vegetable/chicken stock (see recipes on page 58) or use cold water
1 medium sized white onion, chopped
3 garlic cloves, chopped
1½ tsps. cumin
½ tsp. ground cilantro
½ tsp. paprika
1 bay leaf
3 medium carrots, peeled and diced
1 red bell-pepper, diced
2 small red onions, finely sliced
juice of half a lemon
¼ tsp black pepper

SERVES 4

In a large saucepan set over high heat, bring lentils and stock/water to a boil.

Stir in white onion, garlic, spices and bay leaf. Reduce heat to medium/low.

Cover and simmer for 5 minutes.

Stir in the carrots and bell-pepper, cover and simmer for around 15 minutes until the carrots are tender.

Stir in red onion, lemon juice and black pepper.

Cook for a further 10 minutes then serve.

Store any leftovers in an airtight container and refrigerate for up to 3 days or freeze on same day.

PER SERVING:
224 Calories
34g Carbs
13g Protein
4g Fat

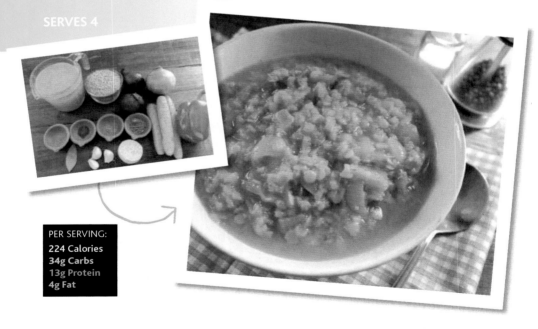

Egg & ham salad

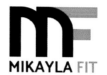

MIKAYLA FIT

2 medium sized eggs
small handful green beans,
ends removed
4 radishes, sliced
handful lettuce leaves
1¾ oz. sliced ham (use
vegetarian ham if preferred *)
8 cherry tomatoes
½ cup cucumber, sliced
2 scallions, chopped
7 olives (optional), sliced
1 tsp. extra virgin olive oil
1 tsp. balsamic vinegar
sprinkle salad seasoning (optional)
see recipe below

SERVES 1

READY IN **10** MINUTES

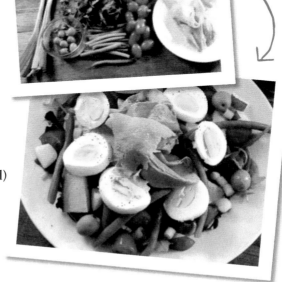

*** Note:** Some meat free alternatives contain gluten and/or MSG. Please check the label before you buy!*

Easy to make salad seasoning:
Lemongrass, Cilantro & Garlic

In a grinder, mix up a teaspoon of dried lemongrass, ground cilantro and garlic powder. Add a pinch of sea salt flakes. Store in an airtight container for future use.

PER SERVING:
340 Calories
16g Carbs
24g Protein
20g Fat

Bring a small pan of salted water to the boil. Add the eggs and simmer gently for 6 minutes. Add the green beans and cook for 4 minutes. then drain. Immerse eggs in cold water for two minutes. Peel eggs and slice.

In a bowl add the lettuce, radishes, ham, eggs, tomatoes, cucumber, cooked beans, olives and scallions.

Drizzle the olive oil and balsamic vinegar onto the salad. Sprinkle with salad seasoning if using.

Store any leftovers in an airtight container and refrigerate for up to 24 hours.

Low carb quiche

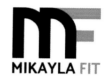

MIKAYLA FIT

a small amount of coconut oil or organic butter to grease tin
2 free range eggs
5 egg whites
½ tsp. black pepper
½ tsp. sea salt flakes
½ tsp. onion powder
½ tsp. Italian seasoning
½ small red onion, finely chopped
½ green bell-pepper, finely chopped
5 cherry tomatoes, halved
1 green chili pepper, finely chopped
handful spinach leaves, chopped
⅓ cup reduced fat grated cheese (optional)

SERVES 2

Preheat oven to 180°C/350°F.

Grease an ovenproof dish or tin (approximately 6 inch square) with coconut oil or butter.

Place all of the ingredients in a large bowl and mix well.

Pour the mixture into the dish and bake for 20-25 minutes, until the center of the quiche is cooked.

Serve with salad.

Store any leftover quiche in an airtight container and refrigerate for up to 24 hours.

PER SERVING:
184 Calories
8g Carbs
20g Protein
8g Fat

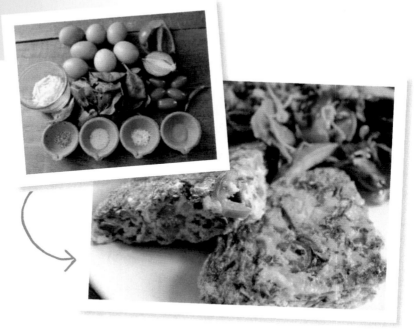

Crunchy mackerel salad

READY IN 10 MINUTES

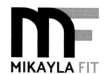

MIKAYLA FIT

handful lettuce leaves
5 cherry tomatoes
1 small stick celery, chopped finely
3 radishes, chopped
⅓ bell-pepper (any color), sliced
¼ cup cucumber, sliced
1 scallion, chopped
4¼ oz. peppered mackerel
1 tsp. extra virgin olive oil
1 tsp. balsamic vinegar
½ tsp. seeds

SERVES 1

Place the lettuce in a bowl. Add the celery, tomatoes, radishes, bell-pepper, cucumber and scallions.

Gently tear the mackerel into large chunks. Add to the salad.

Spoon the olive oil and balsamic vinegar over the salad. Sprinkle with the seeds.

Store any leftovers in an airtight container and refrigerate for up to 24 hours.

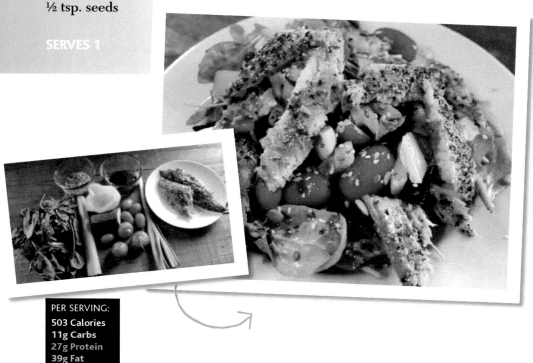

PER SERVING:
503 Calories
11g Carbs
27g Protein
39g Fat

Tomato, basil & carrot soup

MIKAYLA FIT

2 tsps. butter or coconut oil
2 medium sized white onions,
peeled and chopped finely
3 sprigs fresh basil, roughly
chopped plus extra for garnish
3 garlic cloves, peeled and
chopped finely
5 small carrots, peeled and chopped
4 small potatoes, peeled and diced
3 medium sized tomatoes, diced
15¾ fl oz. fresh vegetable stock (see
recipe on page 58) or use 1 organic
stock cube
1 x 400g can chopped tomatoes
Himalayan pink salt plus pepper,
to season

SERVES 4

In a large pan, gently melt the butter or oil.
Add the onions and sauté until soft.

Add the basil and cook for two minutes.
Add the garlic, carrots and potatoes and
cook for 5 minutes.

Add the tomatoes and cook for two
minutes.

Add the stock and canned tomatoes, then
simmer over a gentle heat for 45 minutes.
Remove from heat and allow to cool.

Season well with salt and pepper, then
blend everything in a food processor – just
enough to get the big lumps out.

Serve garnished with finely chopped basil.

*Once cooled, store any leftovers in an
airtight container and refrigerate for up
to 3 days or freeze on same day.*

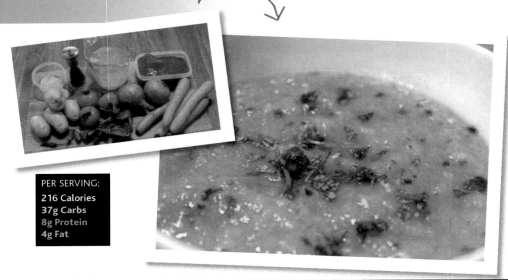

PER SERVING:
216 Calories
37g Carbs
8g Protein
4g Fat

5 veg omelet

3 medium sized eggs plus
1 egg white, beaten
2 tsps. organic butter or coconut oil
2 closed cup mushrooms, sliced
3 medium sized broccoli florets,
finely chopped
¼ red bell-pepper, finely chopped
2 scallions, finely chopped
Himalayan sea salt to season
handful baby leaf spinach, roughly
chopped
2 tsps. low fat hard cheese, grated
(use dairy free cheese if preferred)

SERVES 2

Break the eggs and whites into a jug and beat with a fork and season well.

Melt half of the butter / oil in a non-stick frying pan over a medium heat and add all of the chopped vegetables except for the spinach.

Sauté for 5 minutes, until softened. Remove from heat and set aside.

Remove any bits from the pan. Melt the remaining butter / oil. Pour the eggs into the pan. Cook gently for around 3-4 minutes until the edges of the mixture start to crisp.

When the center of the omelet begins to firm up, add the spinach over the entire omelet. Then carefully add the other vegetables on top of the spinach, so that it wilts. Cook for around 1-2 minutes.

Add the cheese. Using a wooden slice fold the omelet in half. Remove the omelet from the pan and serve.

Once cooled, store any leftovers in an airtight container and refrigerate for up to 24 hours.

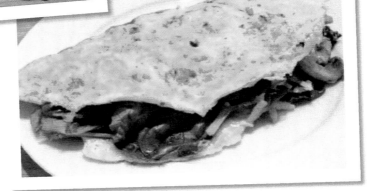

PER SERVING:
210 Calories
4g Carbs
17g Protein
14g Fat

Nourishing mixed bean soup

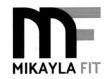

MIKAYLA FIT

2 tsps. organic butter or coconut oil
1 medium sized white onion, finely chopped
3 medium sized carrots, sliced
2 large sticks celery, finely chopped
28¾ oz. chicken breast/meat free chicken*, diced
2 garlic cloves, crushed
1 tsp. paprika
1 tsp. ground cumin
½ tsp. Himalayan pink salt
1 tsp. dried thyme
1 x 400g can chopped tomatoes
1 medium salad tomato, diced
1 Tbsp. tomato purée
16 fl oz. chicken or vegetable stock (see recipes on page 58)
1 red bell-pepper, sliced
7 oz. mixed beans, drained

SERVES 4

*** Note:** *Some meat free alternatives contain gluten and/or MSG. Please check the label before you buy!*

PER SERVING:
290 Calories
16g Carbs
43g Protein
6g Fat

Heat the butter or oil in a large pan. Add the onion and cook gently until softened. Add the carrot and celery and cook for 5 minutes, stirring regularly.

Add the chicken, garlic, spices, salt and thyme. Cook stirring for 10 minutes.

Add the tomatoes, purée, stock and red bell-pepper. Bring to a simmer and cook uncovered for 50 minutes.

Add the mixed beans and cook for a further 5 minutes.

Once cooled, refrigerate for up to 3 days or freeze on the same day.

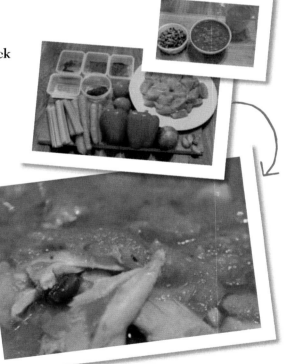

Asian inspired fish salad

3½ oz. white fish
½ a red bell-pepper, diced
½ a yellow bell-pepper, diced
½ a green bell-pepper, diced
few handfuls of lettuce leaves
(optional), torn up into small
pieces
1 tsp. rice vinegar
1 tsp toasted sesame oil
salt and pepper to season

SERVES 1

Bring a saucepan of water to the boil (just enough water to cover the fish).

Reduce to a gentle simmer and place the fish in the water. Cook for 2-3 minutes, turning halfway. When cooked through, remove from heat, drain and leave to cool.

In a salad bowl, mix together the bell-peppers, lettuce (if using) rice vinegar and sesame oil. Break the fish into small pieces, and mix into the salad.

Season well with salt and pepper.

Store in an airtight container and refrigerate for up to 24 hours.

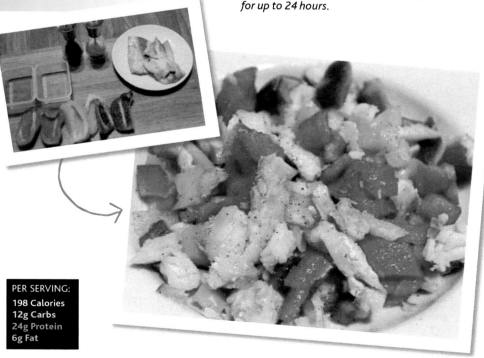

PER SERVING:
198 Calories
12g Carbs
24g Protein
6g Fat

Warming squash & bacon soup

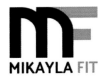

2 tsps. organic butter or coconut oil

2 medium sized white onions, peeled and chopped finely

2 medium sized carrots, peeled and chopped finely

2 garlic cloves, peeled and chopped finely

2 medium sized potatoes, peeled and diced

1 medium sized butternut squash, peeled, deseeded and diced

26¼ fl oz. stock, made with one organic vegetable / chicken stock cube or homemade stock (see recipes on page 58)

1 tsp. dried chili flakes

1 tsp. ground cumin

1 tsp. cilantro powder

salt and pepper to season

4 slices unsmoked back bacon, cut into small pieces

1 small bunch fresh parsley, chopped finely

SERVES 4

PER SERVING:
229 Calories
25g Carbs
12g Protein
9g Fat

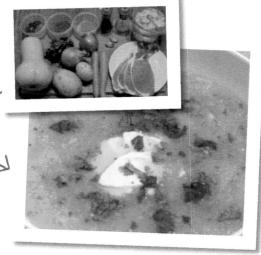

Melt the butter or oil in a large pan over a medium heat. Add the onions and cook, stirring regularly until softened.

Add the carrots and cook for 3 minutes, stirring frequently. Add the garlic and cook for 2 minutes, stirring frequently.

Add the potatoes and butternut squash and stir well, then add the stock, spices, salt and pepper and bacon. Season well. Bring to the boil, then cover and simmer for one hour.

Add a little more water if needed, until the soup is of desired consistency. Add the chopped parsley and cook for a further 10 minutes. Add a dessert spoon of plain yogurt for extra creaminess.

Once cooled, store in an airtight container and refrigerate for up to 3 days or freeze on same day.

Beef, blackberry & kale salad

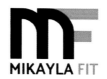

MIKAYLA FIT

1 tsp. coconut oil

1½ Tbsps. tomato purée

1 tsp. fresh garlic, minced

1 tsp. fresh ginger, minced

7 oz. beef rump steaks, cut into strips

1 tsp. garam masala

1 cup kale

½ cup blackberries

READY IN 10 MINUTES

SERVES 1

Melt the oil in a frying pan over a medium heat.

Add the tomato purée, garlic and ginger and stir well to combine.

Add the beef and sprinkle over half of the garam masala. Turn the beef over, and sprinkle on the remaining garam masala.

Cook for 4-5 minutes, until the steak is thoroughly cooked.

Meanwhile, steam the kale gently for 3-4 minutes then drain.

Place the kale on a serving plate and add the blackberries. Top with the cooked beef strips.

Store in an airtight container and refrigerate for up to 24 hours.

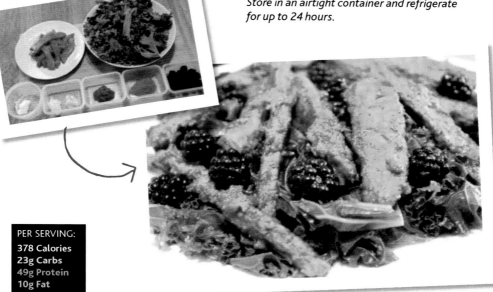

PER SERVING:
378 Calories
23g Carbs
49g Protein
10g Fat

Turkey coconut burgers

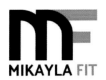

MIKAYLA FIT

26½ oz. lean ground turkey/
vegetarian alternative*
1 small white onion, finely
chopped
1 tsp. sea salt flakes
1 tsp. curry powder
1 tsp. black pepper
1 free range egg
½ a grated coconut
2 cloves garlic, finely chopped
5 green chillies (optional),
finely chopped
3 tsps. organic butter or
coconut oil

MAKES 10 BURGERS

* **Note:** *Some meat free alternatives contain gluten and/or MSG. Please check the label before you buy!*

Top tip:

These also taste great oven baked. Place on a lightly greased tray and cook at 200°C/400°F for 15-20 minutes

Place the mince in a large bowl. Add all of the other ingredients, except for the oil/butter.

Using your hands, mix well for 2-3 minutes. Form into 10 patties and place on a plate.

Melt the oil / butter in a large frying pan over a medium heat. Gently place 5 of the patties in the pan and fry for 15 minutes, turning halfway. Once cooked, fry the other 5 patties.

Serve with a salad and a squeeze of lemon or lime and a plain yoghurt dip.

Store any leftover burgers in an airtight container and refrigerate for up to 3 days.

PER BURGER:
165 Calories
3g Carbs
18g Protein
9g Fat

Spicy green salad

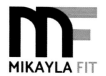

MIKAYLA FIT

2 green chili peppers, finely chopped
1 garlic clove, finely chopped
a small handful of green beans, ends removed
2 tsps. honey
2 Tbsps. fish sauce
2 Tbsps. lime juice
2 tsps. Shaosing rice wine vinegar
a small green papaya or 1 cup cucumber, cut into matchsticks
1 cup carrot, grated
1 Tbsp. roasted peanuts
6 cherry tomatoes, halved

Place the chilis and garlic in a blender and blend well.

Transfer to a large bowl. Add the green beans and pound with a wooden spoon, until they have split.

Add the honey, fish sauce, lime juice and rice wine vinegar. Pound until well combined.

Add the papaya / cucumber, carrot, peanuts and tomatoes and pound gently until the peanuts have broken into small pieces Serve.

Store any leftovers in an airtight container and refrigerate for up to 3 days.

SERVES 1

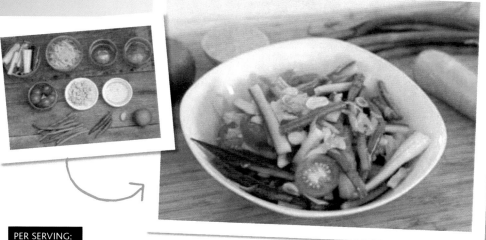

PER SERVING:
375 Calories
55g Carbs
14g Protein
11g Fat

Thai noodle soup

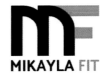

2 tsps organic butter or coconut oil
1 small red onion, sliced
10 kaffir lime leaves
1 red bell-pepper, sliced
½ eggplant, diced
handful mushrooms (any variety), sliced
3 cloves garlic, finely chopped
10½ oz. chicken or turkey breast (cooked or raw), cut into strips
2 Tbsps. red or green Thai cooking paste (choose a low sugar variety)
7 fl oz. coconut milk
15¾ fl oz. fresh chicken stock (see recipe on page 58) or use 1 organic stock cube
handful baby tomatoes
2 Tbsps. fish sauce (nam pla)
2 cups gluten free ribbon rice noodles

SERVES 4

Heat 1 tsp of butter or oil in a large saucepan. Add the onion and sauté for 2-3 minutes. Add the lime leaves, bell-pepper and eggplant, and cook for 3-4 minutes, stirring regularly.

Add the mushrooms and cook for 3 minutes, stirring. Add the garlic, and meat, stir well and cook for 3-4 minutes.

In a small saucepan, melt the remaining butter or oil and add the Thai paste and chicken. Cook for 3 minutes, stirring. Add the coconut milk, stir well and cook for 3 minutes.

Transfer the contents to the large saucepan, add the stock and stir well. Bring to a boil, then reduce to a simmer, stir and cover. Cook for 5 minutes.

Add the tomatoes and fish sauce, stir and cook for 3 minutes. Add the noodles, stir well to separate the strands, and cook for 3 minutes. Serve.

Store any leftovers in an airtight container and refrigerate for up to 2 days or freeze on same day.

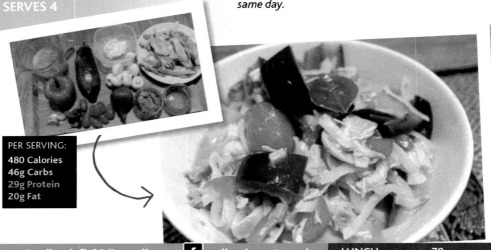

PER SERVING:
480 Calories
46g Carbs
29g Protein
20g Fat

Minty lamb loin with fragrant rice & peas

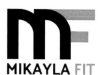

9 oz. lamb loin fillets
2 cloves garlic, finely chopped
a small bunch of fresh mint, finely chopped, plus extra to garnish
a small sprig of rosemary
½ tsp. sea salt
1 Tbsp. butter or coconut oil
½ cup uncooked basmati rice (or use grated cauliflower if preferred)
⅔ cup frozen peas
1 small white onion, finely chopped
grated zest of ½ an unwaxed lemon

SERVES 2

Place the lamb in a large bowl. Add the garlic, mint, rosemary and sea salt. Stir well and cover. Refrigerate for one hour or overnight if you have time.

Preheat oven to 190°C/375°F. Melt half of the butter / oil in a large frying pan. Add the lamb and cook over a medium / high heat for 2 minutes on each side. Finish cooking the lamb for 10 minutes in the oven.

Bring a saucepan of water to the boil and add the rice or cauliflower. Stir well. Reduce heat and simmer until cooked. Remove from water with a slotted spoon and drain. Bring the water back to the boil and add the peas. Reduce heat to simmer and cook for 3-4 minutes. Drain.

Heat the remaining butter / oil in the frying pan and add the onion. Sauté for 2 minutes, stirring. Add the rice and peas to the frying pan and stir well. Cook for 1-2 minutes, stirring. Add the lemon zest to the rice and stir well. Remove pan from heat.

Serve the rice topped with the lamb. Sprinkle the extra chopped mint over the dish and serve.

Consume immediately.

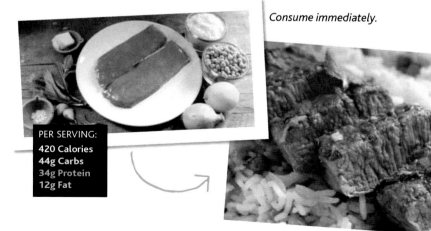

PER SERVING:
420 Calories
44g Carbs
34g Protein
12g Fat

Tomato baked salmon

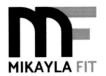

MIKAYLA FIT

1 tsp organic butter or coconut oil
1-2 cloves garlic, finely chopped
½ small red onion, finely chopped
2 vine ripened tomatoes, diced
4 fl oz. chicken or vegetable stock
(see recipes on page 58)
⅙ cup bulgur wheat
2 Tbsps. tomato purée
salt and pepper
1 x 5¼ oz. salmon fillet
handful fresh coriander,
finely chopped
wedge lemon to garnish

SERVES 1

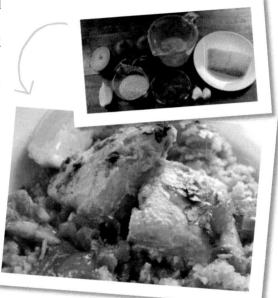

Preheat oven to 150°C/300°F.

In a pan, melt half of the butter or oil over a medium heat. Add the onion and sauté for 3-4 minutes until softened. Add the garlic and sauté for 2-3 minutes, stirring frequently.

Add the tomatoes and cook for 5 minutes.

Add the stock and bring to a steady simmer. Season with salt and pepper and cook for 5 minutes.

Melt the remaining butter or oil in a frying pan over a medium heat. Add the bulgur wheat and gently fry for one minute, stirring frequently.

Pour into an ovenproof dish. Add the tomato mixture and stir well. Add the salmon. Cover loosely with tin foil and cook in the oven for 15-25 minutes, until the salmon is cooked throughout.

Remove from the oven and stir in the coriander. Serve garnished with a wedge of lemon.

Store any leftover salmon in an airtight container and refrigerate for up to 2 days.

PER SERVING:
778 Calories
64g Carbs
54g Protein
34g Fat

Aromatic chicken tagine with apricots

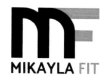

MIKAYLA FIT

2 tsps. butter or coconut oil
21 oz. skinless and boneless chicken thighs
1 white onion, finely chopped
2 garlic cloves, finely chopped
2 inch piece fresh ginger, finely chopped
2 red chili peppers, finely chopped
2 small cinnamon sticks broken into pieces
3 sprigs of fresh rosemary
14 oz. canned peeled plum tomatoes
1½ Tbsps. honey
¾ cup dried pitted apricots
2 Tbsps. flaked almonds
6.75 fl oz. chicken stock (made with one organic stock cube)

SERVES 4

Preheat oven to 180°C/350°F. Melt the butter/oil in a tagine or heavy base casserole dish.

Add the chicken thighs and cook for 1-2 minutes, stirring to brown slightly on both sides.

Add the onion, garlic, ginger, chili peppers, cinnamon sticks and rosemary. Stir well and cook for 5 minutes, allowing the onions to soften.

Add the peeled plum tomatoes, honey, apricots, flaked almonds and chicken stock. Stir well and bring to the boil.

Place the lid on the tagine or casserole dish, transfer to the oven and cook for 50 minutes.

Store any leftovers in an airtight container and refrigerate for up to 3 days or freeze on same day.

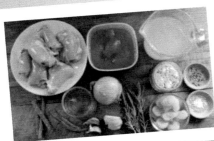

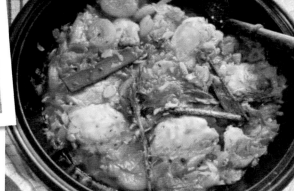

PER SERVING:
486 Calories
37g Carbs
35g Protein
22g Fat

Warming stew

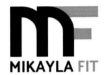

MIKAYLA FIT

1 Tbsp. coconut oil or organic butter
1 small white onion, finely chopped
30oz. lean casserole beef/tofu*, diced
handful closed cup mushrooms, sliced
3 cloves garlic, finely chopped
2 medium sized carrots, peeled and chopped
half a swede, diced
2 cups potatoes, peeled and chopped
2 medium sized parsnips, cut into strips
1 organic stock cube dissolved in 16 fl oz. boiling water
sprig fresh rosemary
1 Tbsp. tomato purée
salt and pepper to season

SERVES 4

Note: Some meat free alternatives contain gluten and/or MSG. Please check the label before you buy!

In a large saucepan, melt the oil or butter over a medium heat. Add the onion, and sauté gently until soft. Transfer to a plate.

Add the beef to the saucepan and brown on all sides (approximately 3-5 minutes), or if using tofu, cook gently for around 4-5 minutes until soft. Transfer to a separate plate.

Add the mushrooms to the saucepan and cook for 3-5 minutes until soft. Add the garlic and cook for two minutes, stirring frequently.

Return the beef/tofu and onions back into the saucepan. Stir in the carrots, swede, parsnips and potatoes and add the stock. There should be enough liquid in the pan to almost cover the vegetables.

Add the rosemary and tomato purée and season well. Cover and simmer for up to two hours (if using beef) or 45 minutes if using tofu. Top up with fresh water if necessary. The sauce will thicken as the potatoes cook.

Once cooled store any leftovers in an airtight container and refrigerate for up to 3 days or freeze on same day.

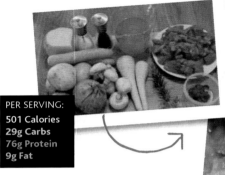

PER SERVING:
501 Calories
29g Carbs
76g Protein
9g Fat

Authentic curry

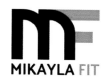

MIKAYLA FIT

1 Tbsp. cumin seeds
1 Tbsp. ghee or coconut oil
5 medium sized onions, diced
5-10 garlic cloves, finely chopped
1-2 inch piece fresh ginger,
peeled and finely chopped
5 green chili peppers, finely chopped
21¼ oz. fresh chicken breast, diced
2 Tbsps. ground turmeric
1 Tbsp. garam masala
1 Tbsp. meat masala
1 Tbsp. sea salt flakes
1 x 400g can chopped tomatoes
1¾ fl oz. cold fresh water
2 Tbsps. per person uncooked
basmati rice
6 florets cauliflower (per person),
finely chopped
handful fresh cilantro, finely
chopped

SERVES 4

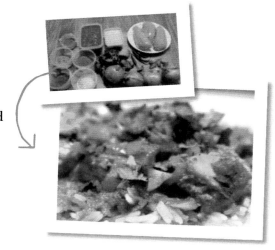

Note: Some meat free alternatives contain gluten and/or MSG. Please check the label before you buy!

PER SERVING:
514 Calories
52g Carbs
54g Protein
10g Fat

In a large pan, roast the cumin seeds gently over a medium heat for 30 seconds. Melt the oil and add the onions. Fry gently for 4 minutes, or until soft. Add the garlic, ginger and chillis. Cook for 1 minute.

Add the chicken, stir and cook for 2 minutes. Add the spices and salt. Stir well, coating the meat in the spices. Add the tomatoes and water and simmer for 10 minutes. Add more water if the mixture becomes dry. Cover and simmer for one hour.

Add the rice to a pan of cold salted water and bring to the boil. Simmer gently until cooked and drain well, reserving the water. Bring the water back to the boil. Add the cauliflower and cook for 2-3 minutes. Drain well. Serve garnished with cilantro.

Store any leftovers in an airtight container and refrigerate for up to 3 days or freeze on same day.

Spaghetti zucchini

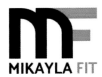

MIKAYLA FIT

2 tsps. organic butter or coconut oil
3 small white onions, finely
chopped
sprig fresh basil leaves and stalks,
chopped roughly
17¾ oz. lean ground beef/
vegetarian alternative*
⅘ cup closed cup mushrooms,
sliced
1 vine-ripened tomato, diced
1 stick celery, finely chopped
½ green bell-pepper, diced
4 cloves garlic, finely chopped
1 x 400g can chopped tomatoes
2 Tbsps. tomato purée
4 large zucchinis
salt and pepper to season

SERVES 4

** **Note:** Some meat free alternatives contain gluten and/or MSG. Please check the label before you buy!*

Heat the butter or oil in a frying pan, over a medium heat. Sauté the onions until soft. Add the chopped basil and fry for 30 seconds. Add the beef and season well with salt and pepper. When the meat is browned, add the mushrooms, vine tomato, celery, bell-pepper and garlic.

Cook gently for 5 minutes. Add the canned tomatoes and purée. Cook over a medium heat for 20 minutes.

Chop the zucchinis into thin spaghetti strips or use a vegetable spiralizer if you have one. Steam gently for 3-4 minutes or until cooked to your liking. Serve.

Once cooled, store any leftover sauce in an airtight container and refrigerate for up to 3 days or freeze on same day.

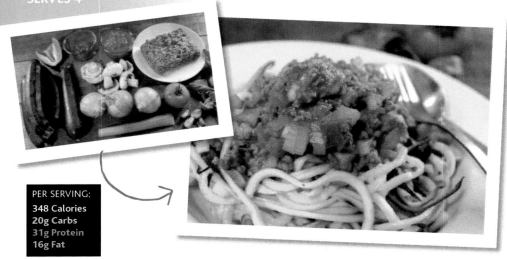

PER SERVING:
348 Calories
20g Carbs
31g Protein
16g Fat

Lentil & sweet potato curry

MIKAYLA FIT

2 tsps. organic butter or coconut oil
12 shallots, chopped
½ tsp. sea salt flakes
2 sweet potatoes, peeled and cut into 1 inch chunks
1 inch piece fresh ginger, peeled and finely chopped
2 small garlic cloves, chopped
1 Tbsp. curry powder
1 bay leaf
17½ fl oz. boiling water
¾ cup red lentils (dry weight)
salt and pepper to season

SERVES 3

Heat the butter or oil in a large saucepan over a gentle heat. Add the shallots and the salt and sauté, stirring occasionally, until the onion softens.

Add the sweet potato, ginger, garlic, curry powder and bay leaf and sauté for one minute until fragrant.

Add the boiling water and stir in the lentils. Reduce the heat to medium / low, cover and simmer for around 18-20 minutes, until the lentils break down and the sweet potatoes are tender.

Season to taste with salt and pepper and serve.

Once cooled, store any leftovers in an airtight container and refrigerate for up to 3 days or freeze on same day.

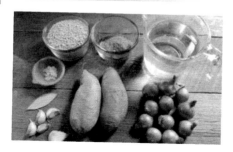

PER SERVING:
235 Calories
44g Carbs
8g Protein
3g Fat

Chicken nuggets

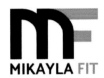

MIKAYLA FIT

1 tsp. coconut flour
1 Tbsp. ground almonds
pinch of paprika
salt and pepper to season
1 tsp. coconut oil
1 medium sized egg
7 oz. fresh chicken breast, diced

MAKES 10 NUGGETS

Preheat the oven to 180°C/350°F.

Mix the flour, almonds, paprika, salt and pepper in a bowl.

In a separate bowl whisk the egg.

Take a piece of chicken and dip it in the egg, coating it evenly. Then dip it in the flour mixture and roll until covered.

Repeat this step with all of the chicken.

Melt the oil in a non stick frying pan over a medium/high heat. Add the chicken and cook for 5 minutes, turning regularly until brown all over.

Transfer the chicken to an oven tray and cook in the oven for 10-15 minutes until cooked through.

Store any leftovers in an airtight container and refrigerate for up to 2 days.

PER NUGGET:
46 Calories
0g Carbs
6g Protein
2g Fat

Chilli con cauli

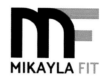

2 tsps. organic butter or coconut oil
2 large white onions, finely chopped
17½ oz. lean ground beef/vegetarian ground beef*
½ green bell-pepper, diced
3 beef tomatoes, diced
5 garlic cloves, finely chopped
4 red or green chili peppers
1 x 400g can chopped tomatoes
1 Tbsp. tomato purée
1 tsp. cayenne pepper
7oz. can kidney beans, drained
¼ cup per person cauliflower, finely chopped or grated
a pinch of sea salt and pepper

SERVES 4

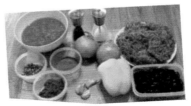

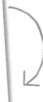

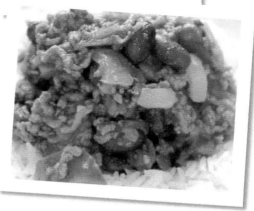

* **Note:** *Some meat free alternatives contain gluten and/or MSG. Please check the label before you buy!*

Heat the butter / oil in a pan over a medium heat and add the onion. Fry for 3-4 minutes, or until soft. Add the mince and cook for 4-5 minutes, stirring to brown all over. Add the salt and pepper.

Add the green pepper and beef tomatoes, and cook for 3-4 minutes, or until soft. Add the garlic cloves and chilli peppers and cook for 1 minute. Add the tinned tomatoes, tomato purée and cayenne pepper. Simmer gently for 15-20 minutes. Add the kidney beans. Cook for 10 minutes.

Bring a pan of cold water to the boil. Add the cauliflower and simmer gently for 3 minutes, or until cooked to your liking. Drain well.

Once cooled, store any leftover chilli sauce in an airtight container and refrigerate for up to 3 days or freeze on same day.

PER SERVING:
365 Calories
36g Carbs
35g Protein
9g Fat

Fragrant fish soup

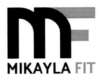

MIKAYLA FIT

3½ fl oz. unsweetened coconut milk

1 Tbsp. fish sauce (nam pla)

juice of one lime

2 Tbsps. soy sauce (or use tamari)

1 tsp. chili flakes

2 tsps. acacia honey

2 Tbsps. per person uncooked basmati rice

2 Tbsps. per person cauliflower, chopped

2 tsps. coconut oil

1 red onion, finely chopped

5-6 cloves garlic, finely chopped

1-2 inch piece fresh ginger, peeled and sliced

1 red chilli, sliced

handful baby carrots, cut into strips

handful shiitake or oyster mushrooms

14 oz. white fish

1 red bell-pepper, sliced

handful beansprouts

SERVES 2

In a small bowl, combine the coconut milk, fish sauce, lime juice, soy sauce, chilli flakes and honey.

Place the rice in a saucepan of boiling water. Reduce to a simmer and cook for 15-20 minutes or until just tender. Add the cauliflower. Cook for 2-3 minutes then drain well.

Place a large saucepan over a medium heat. Add the oil and onion and sauté for 3 minutes. Add the garlic, ginger and chilli and stir fry for 1-2 minutes.

Add the carrot, mushrooms, and half of the sauce. Stir fry for 3 minutes. Add the fish, red pepper, beansprouts and the remaining stir fry sauce. Simmer for 8 minutes, or until the fish is cooked. Add more of the stir fry sauce, to taste.

Store any leftovers in an airtight container and refrigerate for up to 2 days.

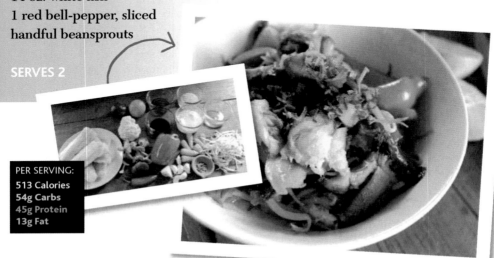

PER SERVING:
513 Calories
54g Carbs
45g Protein
13g Fat

Quick fish stew

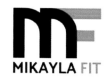

MIKAYLA FIT

2 tsps. organic butter or coconut oil
2 garlic cloves, finely chopped
1½ tsps. ground cumin
1 tsp. paprika
1 tsp. Himalayan salt
8¾ fl oz. cold fresh water
1 x 400g can chopped tomatoes
8 cherry tomatoes
1 green bell-pepper, deseeded and cut into chunks
35¼ oz. white fish fillets, cut into chunks
large handful fresh cilantro, finely chopped
1 lemon, cut into five wedges

SERVES 5

Melt butter or oil in a large saucepan over a medium heat. Add the garlic and stir well. Cook for 30 seconds.

Add the cumin, paprika and salt and cook for one minute, stirring continuously.

Add the water and canned tomatoes. Bring to the boil, then reduce to a simmer. Add the bell-pepper, and simmer for 5 minutes.

Add the fish and cherry tomatoes and cook for 10 minutes until the fish falls apart. Break the fish up with a wooden spoon.

Stir in the cilantro and remove from heat. Serve with a wedge of lemon.

Store any leftovers in an airtight container and refrigerate for up to 3 days or freeze on same day.

Suggestion:

Tastes great with a serving of fresh green leafy vegetables, such as spinach or kale

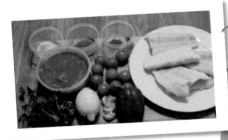

PER SERVING:
253 Calories
6g Carbs
46g Protein
5g Fat

Low carb chilli cheese burgers

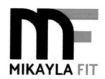
MIKAYLA FIT

8¾ oz. lean ground beef/vegetarian
alternative*)
1 tsp. chili powder
½ tsp. sea salt flakes
1 tsp. black pepper
½ small white onion, very finely
chopped
1 egg
3 tsps. organic butter or coconut oil
4 large portobello mushrooms
¼ cup hard cheese, cut into slices
(use dairy free cheese if preferred)
1 large beef tomato, sliced
3 tsps. low sugar relish sauce
(optional)
handful fresh spinach leaves,
chopped

SERVES 2

*** Note:** *Some meat free alternatives contain gluten and/or MSG. Please check the label before you buy!*

Place the beef in a large bowl and gently pound it with a wooden spoon to break it up into small pieces. Add the chili powder, salt, pepper and onion and mix well.

Add the egg and mix for 2-3 minutes with your hands until the mixture is well combined. Shape the mixture into two patties and place them on a plate.

RECIPE CONTINUED ON NEXT PAGE >>

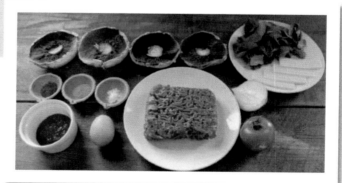

PER SERVING:
393 Calories
11g Carbs
40g Protein
21g Fat

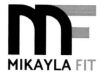

MIKAYLA FIT

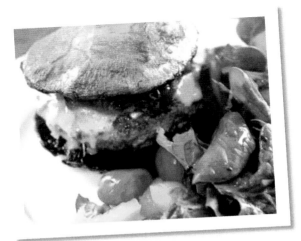

Melt the butter or oil in a saucepan, remove from heat and brush half of the butter onto both sides of the mushrooms. Place the mushrooms on a foil lined grill tray.

Place the saucepan over a medium heat. When the butter or oil starts to bubble, add the burgers. Cook for 6 minutes then turn over carefully with a slice and cook for a further 5 minutes. Remove from heat.

Meanwhile, prepare a hot grill. Place the mushrooms under the grill and reduce heat to medium. Grill for 5 minutes each side or until soft. Add the cheese slices to the burgers then place under the grill for several minutes, until the cheese has melted.

Place one mushroom on a plate, top side down. Add a burger patty, then a slice or two of tomato, followed by half of the relish (if using) and then top with spinach. Add another mushroom, rounded side up to complete the burger.

Repeat the process again to create the second burger. Serve with a leafy green salad.

Store any leftover burger patties in an airtight container and refrigerate for up to 3 days or freeze on same day.

Mediterranean salmon & cod bake

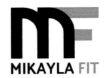

MIKAYLA FIT

1 zucchini, chopped
1 medium red onion, chopped
2 garlic cloves, finely chopped
13 cherry tomatoes, halved
2 bell-peppers (any colour),
chopped
2 Tbsps. extra virgin olive oil
2 Tbsps. balsamic vinegar
10oz. fresh salmon fillets
10oz. fresh cod loin
1 tsp. dried Italian herbs
a pinch of salt and pepper

SERVES 3

Preheat the oven to 180°C/350°F.

Place the zucchini, garlic, onion, peppers and cherry tomatoes on a large baking tray and spread them out evenly.

Sprinkle the olive oil and balsamic vinegar over the vegetables. Bake for 10 minutes.

Remove the tray from the oven and nestle the salmon and cod amongst the vegetables. **Note:** If the salmon fillets are a much thicker cut than the cod, cut the salmon into chunks so that it cooks at around the same rate as the cod.

Sprinkle the Italian herbs, salt and pepper over everything. Bake for around 25 minutes or until the fish is cooked thoroughly.

Store any leftovers in an airtight container and refrigerate for up to 1 day.

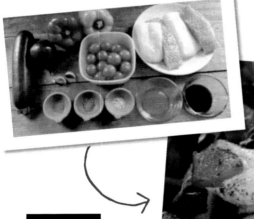

PER SERVING:
398 Calories
13g Carbs
38g Protein
22g Fat

Spinach & cheese pizza

small amount of coconut
oil/ or butter to grease dish
4 medium sized eggs
3 egg whites
⅔ cup porridge oats (use gluten free
oats if preferred)
4 cherry tomatoes, halved
1½ cups baby leaf spinach, finely
chopped
1 red chili pepper, finely chopped
½ green bell-pepper, finely chopped
1 tsp. paprika
1 tsp. dried oregano
3 Tbsps. low fat soft cream cheese
(use dairy free cheese if preferred)
salt and pepper to season

MAKES 6 SLICES

Suggestion:

This recipe tastes great either warm
from the oven or straight from the
fridge. Makes a great portable snack.

Preheat oven to 150°C/300°F.

Lightly grease a large round ovenproof dish
with coconut oil or butter.

Whisk the eggs and egg whites in a jug.
Season well.

Add the oats, vegetables, dried spices and
herbs and stir well.

Pour into the dish and cook for around 10
minutes, until center of mixture is cooked.

Spoon on the cheese, and cook for a
further 5 minutes.

*Store any leftovers in an airtight container
and refrigerate for up to 2 days.*

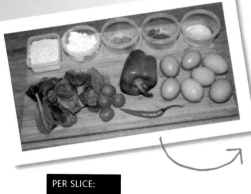

PER SLICE:
93 Calories
6g Carbs
9g Protein
4g Fat

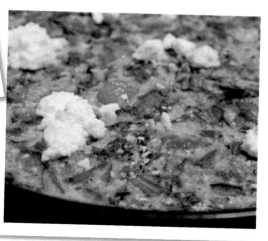

Hearty chicken casserole

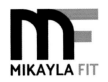

1 Tbsp. ghee or coconut oil

2lb 3 oz. skinless boneless chicken thighs

a good pinch of sea salt and ground black pepper

1 small white onion, chopped

2 garlic cloves, finely chopped

2 celery sticks, sliced

2 cups carrots, peeled and sliced

1 large leek, sliced

2 cups white potatoes, peeled and diced

1 Tbsp. plain flour (use gluten free if preferred)

26.5 fl oz. hot chicken stock (made with one organic stock cube)

1 bouquet garni (available in major supermarkets)

⅓ cup uncooked quinoa (optional)

SERVES 4

Heat the ghee/oil in a large saucepan over a medium heat. Season the chicken with salt and pepper. Place in the pan and fry gently for 5 minutes on each side. Transfer to a plate and set aside.

Drain most of the excess fat from the saucepan. Add the onion, garlic, celery, carrots, leek and potatoes and fry for 5 minutes, stirring occasionally.

Stir in the flour and cook for 1 minute. Add the stock and bouquet garni.

Bring to a simmer and add the chicken. Stir gently, ensuring the chicken is covered in the liquid. Cover and simmer for 15 minutes.

Rinse the quinoa (if using) and drain well. Add it to the saucepan. Stir well and simmer for 25 minutes. Taste and add more seasoning, if required. Remove the bouquet garni and discard. Serve.

Store any leftovers in an airtight container and refrigerate for up to 4 days or freeze on same day.

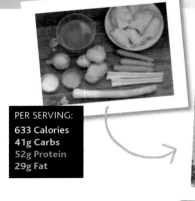

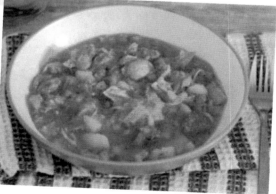

PER SERVING:
633 Calories
41g Carbs
52g Protein
29g Fat

Peruvian chicken

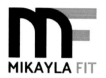

2 tsps. coconut oil
19.5 oz. chicken breast, finely chopped
1 small white onion, chopped
1 cup carrot, peeled and chopped
2 garlic cloves, chopped
2 tsps. fresh ginger, finely chopped
1-2 tsps. chili powder
2 tsps. ground cumin
½ tsp. ground red chili flakes
1 tsp. soy sauce or tamari
juice of 1 lime
a pinch of sea salt and ground black pepper
1-2 Tbsps. fresh cilantro, finely chopped

SERVES 3

Heat the oil in a large saucepan. Add the chicken and fry gently for 6-8 minutes, or until cooked. Transfer to a plate and set aside.

Add the onion and carrot to the saucepan. Cook for 4-5 minutes, stirring occasionally.

Add the garlic and ginger and cook for around 3 minutes, stirring occasionally.

Add the chicken back into the pan, along with the chili powder, cumin, chili flakes, soy sauce, lime juice, salt and pepper.

Stir well and cook for 5 minutes, stirring occasionally. Serve garnished with fresh cilantro.

Store any leftovers in an airtight container and refrigerate for up to 4 days or freeze on same day.

Serving suggestion:

Serve on a bed of steamed rice and / or leafy greens

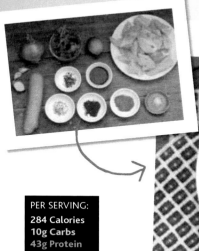

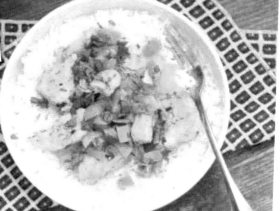

PER SERVING:
284 Calories
10g Carbs
43g Protein
8g Fat

Spicy Thai burgers

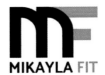

MIKAYLA FIT

For the burgers:
15¾ oz. lean ground turkey/
vegetarian alternative*
1 medium sized egg
small bunch fresh cilantro, finely
chopped,
plus extra to garnish
1 green chilli, finely sliced
2 scallions, finely sliced
1 tsp. Thai 7 Spice seasoning
half a small red onion, finely chopped
slice of fresh lime to garnish

For the vegetable side dishes:
2 large sweet potatoes
1 tsp. ground cinnamon
10 cherry tomatoes, sliced in half
2 cups baby leaf spinach

MAKES 5 BURGERS AND
3 SERVINGS OF MASH AND VEG

*Note: Some meat free alternatives contain
gluten and/or MSG. Please check the label
before you buy!*

Preheat oven to 175°C/350°F.

In a large bowl, mash up the turkey,
using a masher or your hands. Add the
remaining burger ingredients and mix well
until well combined. Shape the mixture
into 5 patties, then transfer to a lightly
greased baking tray. Oven cook for 10
minutes. Turn over and cook for a 10-15
minutes. The juices will run clear when
cooked.

For the vegetable side dishes: Bake the
sweet potatoes in the oven for 45 minutes
or until soft. Using a fork, scrape the
contents of the potatoes into a bowl.
Discard the skin. Mash thoroughly and
season well. Stir in the cinnamon.

Pour cold water into a non-stick frying pan
(just enough to cover the base). Add the
tomatoes and cook gently for 2 minutes,
stirring frequently. Add the spinach and
wilt gently.

*Store the burgers and mash in separate
airtight containers and refrigerate for up to
3 days.*

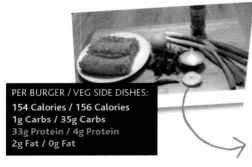

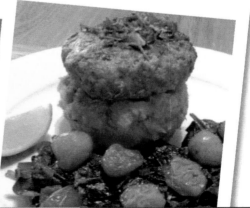

PER BURGER / VEG SIDE DISHES:
154 Calories / 156 Calories
1g Carbs / 35g Carbs
33g Protein / 4g Protein
2g Fat / 0g Fat

Lime chicken fajitas

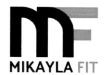
MIKAYLA FIT

IDEAL FOR BBQ

17¾ oz. chicken breast/
vegetarian chicken*, diced
juice of 2 limes
4 cloves garlic, finely chopped
2 tsps. coconut oil or butter
1 red bell-pepper, diced
1 green bell-pepper, diced
1 yellow bell-pepper, diced
1 medium sized white onion,
finely sliced
½ tsp. ground cumin
¼ tsp. sea salt flakes
¼ tsp. ground black pepper
pre-soaked wooden skewers

SERVES 3

Note: Some meat free alternatives contain gluten and/or MSG. Please check the label before you buy!

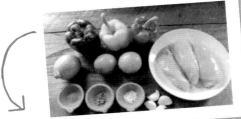

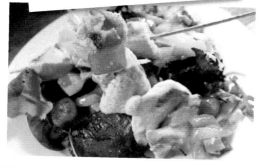

Put the chicken in a bowl. Combine the lime juice and about half of the garlic. Pour the mixture over the chicken, coating thoroughly. Cover the dish and allow it to marinate in the refrigerator for up to 30 minutes. Any longer and the lime juice will break down too much of the tissue.

Preheat the oven to 150°C/300°F or prepare the barbecue for cooking.

PER SERVING:
358 Calories
13g Carbs
54g Protein
10g Fat

Remove chicken from fridge and thread several chicken pieces onto each skewer. Place the chicken on the barbecue or in the oven and turn regularly until cooked through (around 20 minutes).

Heat the oil in a large skillet over a medium heat. Add the bell-peppers, onion and remaining garlic to the skillet. Cook for around five minutes or until tender, stirring regularly. Sprinkle with cumin, salt and pepper. Serve the fajita mix and chicken with a side salad.

Store any leftover chicken in an airtight container and refrigerate for up to 3 days.

Lime & ginger pork meatballs

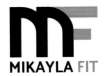

MIKAYLA FIT

14 oz. 10% fat ground pork
a small handful of fresh
cilantro, finely chopped
1 Tbsp. soy sauce (or tamari
sauce)
1 tsp. Chinese five spice
1 inch thick piece of fresh
ginger, grated
grated zest of ½ a lime
2 tsps. coconut oil
1 cup Tenderstem broccoli or
broccoli, roughly chopped
1 red bell-pepper, roughly
chopped
2 cloves garlic, finely sliced
1 small red onion, sliced
1 medium sized carrot, sliced

SERVES 2

Preheat the oven to 210°C/425°F.

Place the pork in a large bowl. Add the cilantro, soy sauce, Chinese five spice, ginger and lime zest.

Using your hands, mix the ingredients together and form 10 meatballs.

Place the meatballs on an oven tray and bake for 20-25 minutes, until cooked.

Melt the coconut oil in a wok over a high temperature. Add the vegetables and garlic and stir fry for 4-5 minutes or until the vegetables are cooked to your liking.

Arrange the meatballs over the vegetables. Serve.

Store any leftover meatballs in an airtight container and refrigerate for up to 3 days or freeze on same day. Store any leftover vegetables in an airtight container and refrigerate for up to 2 days.

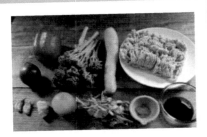

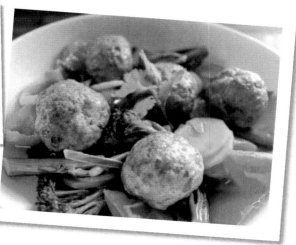

PER SERVING:
392 Calories
10g Carbs
43g Protein
20g Fat

Lamb curry

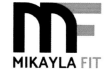
MIKAYLA FIT

4 medium tomatoes
1 Tbsp. coconut oil or butter
1 bay leaf
5 green cardamom pods
1 large white onion, finely diced
24¾ oz. lean lamb, diced
1 thumb-sized piece of fresh
ginger, peeled and roughly chopped
8-10 garlic cloves, peeled and
roughly chopped
1 tsp. turmeric
2 tsps. cilantro powder
1 tsp. garam masala
1 tsp. sea salt flakes
3-4 green chili peppers, finely
chopped
7 fl oz. cold fresh water
½ cup per person, cauliflower
handful fresh cilantro,
finely chopped

SERVES 4

Carefully immerse the tomatoes in a saucepan of recently boiled water.

Meanwhile, melt the oil/butter in a large saucepan. Add the bay leaf and cardamom pods and fry for 30 seconds. Add the onion and fry for 4 minutes, or until softened. Add the lamb, and fry for 4-5 minutes, stirring regularly.

In a blender, mix the ginger and garlic with a splash of cold water. Add the mixture to the lamb, along with the spices, salt and chillis. Cook for 2-3 minutes, stirring regularly.

RECIPE CONTINUED ON NEXT PAGE >>

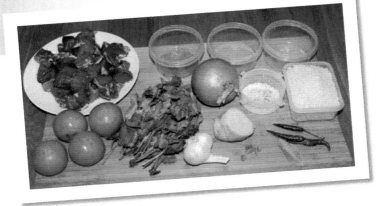

PER SERVING:
398 Calories
21g Carbs
56g Protein
10g Fat

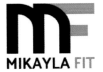
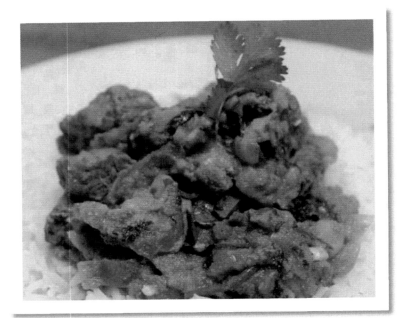

Remove the tomatoes from the water and carefully peel off the skin.Mash thoroughly in a bowl.

Add the tomatoes to the lamb. Simmer for 10 minutes. Add the water and bring to a boil. Cover and reduce heat to simmer. Cook for 45 minutes, stirring occasionally. Add more water if the curry becomes dry.

10 minutes before the end of cooking time, bring a saucepan of water to the boil. Add the cauliflower and cook for 2-3 minutes. Drain well.

Serve the curry garnished with cilantro.

Store any leftovers in an airtight container and refrigerate for up to 3 days or freeze on same day.

Easy lamb stew

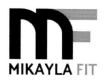

2 tsps. ghee or coconut oil
2 cups white onion, finely chopped
2¼ cups carrot, peeled and sliced
17.75 oz. stewing lamb, visible fat removed, diced
2 cloves garlic, finely chopped
1 sprig fresh rosemary
17 fl oz. lamb or vegetable stock, made with one organic stock cube
2 cups potatoes, peeled and diced
salt and pepper to season

SERVES 4

Melt the ghee / oil in a large saucepan over a medium heat. Add the onion and sauté gently for 3-4 minutes, stirring.

Add the carrot and sauté for 3-4 minutes, stirring occasionally.

Add the lamb, stir well and cook for 4 minutes. Stir occasionally to seal on all sides.

Add the garlic and rosemary and fry gently for 2 minutes, stirring.

Add the potatoes and stock and stir well. Season with salt and pepper. Bring to the boil then reduce to a simmer. Cover and cook for 30 minutes.

If the mixture is too dry or thick, add some boiling water. Stir well and cook for one hour, or until the lamb is tender (checking the thickness of the stew halfway through cooking time).

Store any leftovers in an airtight container and refrigerate for up to 3 days or freeze on same day.

Serving suggestion:

Serve with steamed greens of your choice.

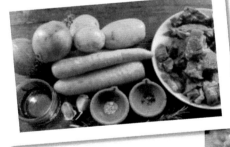

PER SERVING:
465 Calories
30g Carbs
30g Protein
25g Fat

Cauliflower cheese bake

1 tsp. coconut oil or butter

2 medium sized leeks, chopped

1 cup cauliflower, grated

7 fl oz. fresh chicken or vegetable stock (see recipe on page 58)

15 baby plum tomatoes

⅔ cup frozen peas

1-2 green chili peppers

½ tsp. black pepper

½ tsp. sea salt flakes

½ tsp. paprika

½ tsp. Italian herb mix

⅘ cup hard cheese, grated (use dairy free cheese if preferred)

SERVES 2

Melt the oil / butter in a large frying pan over a medium heat.

Add the leeks and cauliflower. Sauté for 3-4 minutes, stirring frequently.

Add the stock and mix well. Add the tomatoes, peas and chilis.

Add the salt, pepper, spices and herbs. Sauté until everything starts to soften. Add more stock if the base of the pan becomes dry during cooking.

Remove pan from heat.

Prepare a medium / hot grill.

Spoon a layer of the mixture into an ovenproof dish (or use several smaller dishes if preferred). Add a layer of cheese then another layer of vegetable mixture. Top with the remaining cheese.

Grill for around 3 minutes, or until the cheese is golden and bubbling.

Consume immediately.

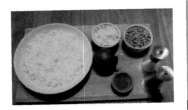

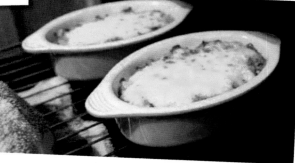

PER SERVING:
334 Calories
22g Carbs
21g Protein
18g Fat

Made in the USA
Middletown, DE
23 September 2023

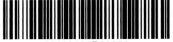

39169120R00075